THE GUIDE TO TRAVELING GLUTEN FREE

Learn how to find safe, gluten-free food options on your next travel adventure

ELIKQITIE

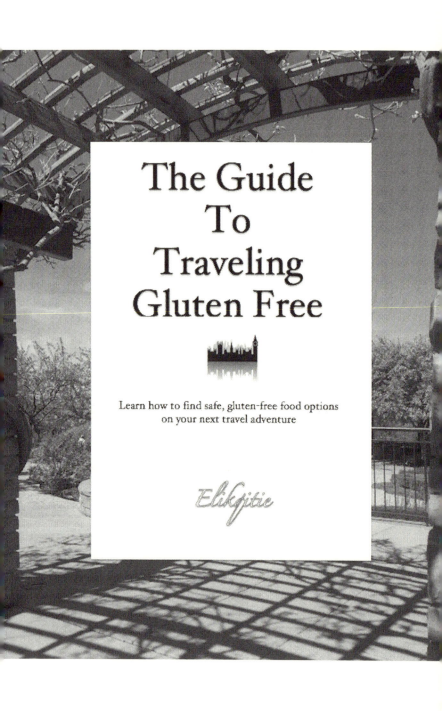

The Guide To Traveling Gluten Free

Learn how to find safe, gluten-free food options on your next travel adventure

Elikjitie

Copyright © 2020 by Travel Gluten Free, LLC
The Guide to Traveling Gluten Free
All rights reserved. No part of this publication may be reproduced, distributed or transmitted in any form, including photocopying, recording, or other electronic or mechanical methods, without the prior written permission of the author, except in the case of brief quotations embodied in critical reviews and certain other noncommercial uses permitted by copyright law.

Although the author has made every effort to ensure that the information in this book was correct at press time, the author and publisher do not assume and hereby disclaim any liability to any party for any loss, damage, or disruption caused by errors or omissions, whether such errors or omissions result from negligence, accident, or any other cause.

Adherence to all applicable laws and regulations, including international, federal, state and local governing professional licensing, business practices, advertising, and all other aspects of doing business in the US, Canada, or any other jurisdiction is the sole responsibility of the reader and consumer. Author does not assume any responsibility or liability whatsoever on behalf of the consumer or reader of this material. Any perceived slight of any individual or organization is purely unintentional.

Resources in this book are provided for informational purposes only and should not be used to replace the specialized training and professional judgment of a healthcare professional. The author cannot be held responsible for the use of the information provided within this book. Please always consult a trained professional before making any decision regarding treatment of yourself or others.

ISBN: 9781735587806

All photographs were taken by Elikqitie and are sole property of Travel Gluten Free, LLC

Ziploc is a registered trademark of SC Johnson.

Available for special quantity discounts to organizations.

Please contact Elikqitie on the Contact page on our website at www.travelglutenfreepodcast.com

Travel Gluten Free, LLC
6300 Sagewood Dr.
STE H216
Park City, Utah, 84098

YOUR FREE EBOOK

Most Visited Gluten Free Cities in America

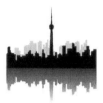

Looking to get your hands on more great gluten-free travel information? Then download my free e-book, Most Visited Gluten Free Cities in America with over 30 pages of information for even more travel resources!

You'll find a local tourism link to view fun activities for each city listed, and, of course, highly delicious dedicated and gluten-free friendly restaurants that are celiac-safe along with restaurant location and phone numbers for each of the establishments listed in this vacation guide.

Get your free eBook now as a Thank You for purchasing The Guide to Traveling Gluten Free!
bit.ly/3gvq8y7

ARE YOU LISTENING?

Listen in to the Travel Gluten Free Podcast With Elikqitie!

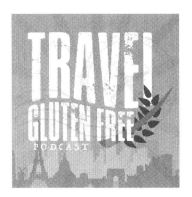

Travel Gluten Free is the leading podcast for anyone leading a gluten-free lifestyle and looking for a better way to live your gluten-free life. Don't settle for just living your gluten-free lifestyle; love your gluten-free lifestyle!

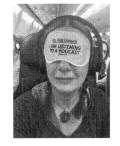

Find exciting new foods, foods that travel well, and gluten-free travel advice from Elikqitie along with great resources to use when traveling and eating gluten-free every day.

CONTENTS

Meet the Author	xi
1. You Just Found Out You Can't Eat "Normal" Bread, Now What?	1
2. Gluten Free Foods and Certified Gluten Free Foods: What's the Difference?	11
3. The Challenge: Eating Out Gluten-Free	20
4. How to Plan Ahead and Be Ready for Gluten Free Travel	38
5. Using Gluten Free Apps to Shop for Safe Food	44
6. Stores that Offer Gluten Free Foods	48
7. How to Avoid Gluten While Traveling	55
8. Supplements You Can Travel with When You're Gluten-Free	59
9. So You've Been Glutened, Now What?	75
10. Gluten Free Travel Cosmetics	80
11. How to Pack Your Gluten Free Travel Bags	88
12. Travel By Air	93
13. Gluten Free Road Trips	111
14. Camping Gluten-Free	117
15. Cruising Gluten Free	129
16. Top Ten Gluten Free Friendly Cities in America	144
17. Traveling Gluten Free in National Parks	166
18. Travel Abroad	179
Work With Me	197
Share This Book with the World!	199

INTRODUCTION

Are you anxious about traveling with Celiac Disease? Does the thought of getting sick on vacation worry you to no end? Unsure of what travel options are safe and how to choose a safe restaurant away from home for you and your children?

The Guide to Traveling Gluten Free will walk you through the process of planning and enjoying your next gluten-free travel adventure! Take the guesswork out of how to travel, where to go, and how to eat safely when you follow the information in my guide. Whether you are Celiac or gluten intolerant, my guide will give you handy information to delight in your next vacation experience!

Learn how to take a trip safely, what questions to ask when you are at a restaurant and which online tools and apps to utilize to find safe, dedicated gluten-free restaurants and food options. Find out what stores to shop at to purchase gluten-free food, determine if a restaurant is gluten-free or celiac friendly, and when you should walk out of a restaurant.

Become competent in choosing, packing, and traveling with delicious and safe snacks on your next flight. Acquaint yourself with the steps to plan your vacation, plan easy camping food, and handle the packing and bringing food with you on your next road trip.

Being a lover of food and avid traveler, I found out how the added complexities of being gluten-free and the anxiety of getting sick while on your excursion can put a damper on your recreation and adventure. After driving over 6,000 miles of road trips, taking dozens of flights, and experiencing several cruises on multiple cruise lines, I found out what actions and words worked, and how to implement them in advance of my trip to ensure I always have safe eating options.

When you move through The Guide to Traveling Gluten Free, I'll walk you step-by-step through travel planning, no matter where you want to go or what you want to do.

I've used the information procured in my guide on numerous cruises, road trips, and adventures! From southern Utah to Philadelphia, to Austria, Norway, London, and Iceland, the information in this guide is what I've used and continue to apply to safely eat while traveling the world. The only time I've been glutened on a trip was when I didn't follow one of the steps in my Guide to Traveling Gluten Free.

You and your gluten-free entourage can now eat safely while you voyage, without the worry of accidental contamination. With my guide, you will be able to ascertain avoidable situations concerning cross-contaminated food. Experience carefree adventures on your next trip when you use the advice in The Guide to Traveling Gluten Free.

How will you plan your next gluten-free adventure? When do you need to start? Start by picking up the The Guide to Traveling Gluten Free to jumpstart your next vacation. Plan now to enjoy your next vacation as soon as possible! Collect your ideas and develop your sightseeing plans now for your next vacation retreat!

Love *The Guide to Traveling Gluten Free?* Then I invite you to tune in for more travel advice, learn about exciting new gluten-free products, and find out the best activities in different cities by watching my YouTube Channel and listening to my podcast Travel Gluten Free. Found on your favorite podcast player, including Apple Podcasts, Pandora, Stitcher, Overcast, Himalaya and Google Podcasts, learn how to Enjoy Food, Enjoy Travel and Enjoy Life!

Elikqitie

DEDICATION

This book is dedicated to everyone in our gluten-free community who seek the freedom to travel and live their life checking off their bucket list items without reserve.

My work is also dedicated to my two wonderful daughters, Anabelle and Aliyah who have kept me going in the downtimes and who I can always count on to brighten my day and bring a smile to my face.

MEET THE AUTHOR

A native of Philadelphia, Elikqitie grew up eating the staple cultural foods of her native city, such as cheesesteaks, Tastycakes, and soft pretzels. While Celiac Disease has changed her eating habits a bit, she is still a foodie at heart!

While living the gluten-free lifestyle can be quite challenging, Elikqitie takes on these challenges to continue to live her life, enjoying travel, and exploring delectable new foods. Her love of travel mixed with her continual drive for staying on the cutting edge of health has led her to blend her passion and creativity in publishing her podcast "Travel Gluten Free." By combining great interviews and informational monologue, she shares her "how-to" for living a gratifying, gluten-free life. She loves to share her knowledge and experience with our gluten-free community.

Elikqitie is based in Park City, UT, within driving distance to the world's largest ski resort and five of the most beautiful National Parks the US has to offer! She loves frolicking in the outdoors and enjoys skiing, hiking, camping, mountain biking, and the multitude of outdoor activities Utah offers. 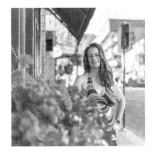 Her central location in the US provides many opportunities to travel to magnificent places where she discovers new gluten-free bakeries, products, and extraordinary people

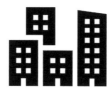

www.travelglutenfreepodcast.com

Find me on Youtube, Tumblr, and other social platforms.

- facebook.com/travelglutenfreepodcast
- twitter.com/TravelGFMe
- instagram.com/travelglutenfreepodcast
- pinterest.com/travelglutenfree

❧ 1 ☙

YOU JUST FOUND OUT YOU CAN'T EAT "NORMAL" BREAD, NOW WHAT?

Many of us love foods that contain gluten. When we find out we need to eliminate gluten from our diet, our minds immediately turn to the absence of bread in our lives. Then we think about other foods we are so fond of, which contain gluten such as pasta, cereal, and baked goods. If you're a beer drinker, that's out too - unless you purchase gluten-free beer or gluten-free hard cider.

Then it hits you like a brick wall, and you realize that you can't eat gluten again. All of your most beloved treats and essential food items have been ripped from your existence - forever!

You feel like your best friend telling you that the Zombie Apocalypse is scheduled for tomorrow at dawn would be less of a burden than giving up your beloved gluten. But what is gluten, and what foods do I really need to avoid when taking gluten out of my diet?

In actuality, you don't have to take many of the foods you like to eat out of your diet. You do, however, need to try gluten-free versions of those foods. Gluten-free food, similar to gluten-containing foods, have brands that are good and brands that aren't so good. Eating gluten-free doesn't mean giving up what you love, but finding a different way to enjoy that food!

If you're Celiac, this means giving up gluten for the rest of your life. Remember, you are treating disease, not a "stomach ache." In many cases, giving up gluten if you have an autoimmune disease will yield a healthier you. Many people I've talked to with Hashimoto's disease, Graves, Lupus, and Rheumatoid Arthritis usually see a remarkable difference in their health when eating gluten-free.

WHAT IS GLUTEN?

Gluten is a protein found in different types of grains, including wheat, spelt, Kamut, einkorn, faro, barley, rye, and triticale.

Many people who are not gluten-free or new to being gluten-free are not sure what grains they can and cannot eat. Here is a list of grains (in alphabetical order) containing gluten that you want to avoid if you are trying out gluten-free or have an autoimmune condition such as Celiac disease.

The following is a list of grains that contain gluten and common everyday foods these grains are found. Always note: gluten can hide in many different places other than this list. Make sure to read through to the end of this chapter to find out where gluten hides. Oh yes, and ALWAYS read the ingredients list - don't trust the label that says "gluten-free." There have been products on shelves for consumers to purchase that read "gluten-free" and are improperly labeled.

BARLEY

Barley is commonly found in malt, malt flavoring, malt extract, malted milk products, malted barley, barley flour, malt syrup, malt vinegar. Ingredients listed as malt are most likely going to be created from barley, with very few exceptions. One of which is gluten-free beer made from grains other than barley or hops.

- food coloring can contain barley
- barley is added to soups as a main ingredient i.e., barley soup
- beer is commonly made from barley grain
- brewer's Yeast

Rye

Rye can be found mainly in bread, but can also be found in other foods. Rye has a distinctive taste and is commonly found in:

- bread
- cereals
- croutons

Spelt

Spelt differs from wheat as the gluten in spelt has a different molecular make-up than wheat gluten. Spelt has more fiber, as a result, is more water-soluble. Modern wheat has been hybridized to contain twenty times (yes, that is NOT a typo) more gluten content. This is what we are eating in our commercial baked goods. Spelt flour is used in:

- pasta
- cookies

- crackers
- cakes
- Muffins
- cereals
- pancakes
- waffles

TRITICALE

Triticale is a newer grain, hybridized from crossing wheat and rye, known as a fodder crop. While widely used as feed for animals, you can find this crop in people food too. Triticale is most commonly found in different breakfast cereals, but can also frequently be found in bread and pasta. Make sure to read the ingredients label and not consume foods with triticale if you have an issue with gluten. Triticale is commonly found in the same types of foods that wheat is found.

WHEAT

Today, our modern wheat is hybridized to contain twenty times more gluten. Additionally, wheat is sprayed with a variety of chemicals for maturation and other production purposes. The wheat we eat today is not your grandma's wheat. Between hybridization and the number of chemicals sprayed on wheat, your grandma wouldn't recognize the process that this popular grain runs through before eating it. Wheat is commonly found in:

- bread
- used in gravies as a thickener
- waffles, pancakes and other breakfast items

- baked goods
- used in soups as a thickener
- pasta
- cereals, the main ingredient of many cereals is wheat
- sauces such as BBQ sauce, roux and other sauces placed on meats and
- vegetables
- salad dressings
- marinades for meats and vegetables
- croutons
- tortillas
- truffle candy

Wheat derivatives which also contain gluten:

- durum wheat
- semolina, a popular flour
- spelt
- In cereal in the form of wheat farina
- faro, an ancient grain, found in risottos, salads, and cereals
- graham as in graham crackers
- einkorn wheat

PLACES GLUTEN LIKES TO HIDE

Gluten is sneaky, yes, sneaky. You can find gluten in many unexpected places you wouldn't think to look. For someone who is eliminating gluten to see if not eating gluten is going to make a difference health-wise, this may not be a huge concern. For those of us who have Celiac disease, hidden gluten is similar to that scary character in a horror film that everyone trusts. The entire movie you think this character is doing good, only to find out this is the same character who has been killing everyone in the film. If you have Celiac disease, that is precisely what gluten does when you consume gluten. This protein kills you off slowly, little by little, by decimating the tissue in your small intestine that absorbs nutrients in your body.

Always suspect the following foods will contain gluten. Actually, I suspect that every food which I see at the grocery store has gluten, even if the bag says "Gluten-Free" on the front. These labels hold no power unless the label specifically says "Certified Gluten-Free" which we will get into later in this book.

These are foods and other places which I have found gluten "hiding" in unexpectedly:

- rice cereal
- soy sauce
- salted peanuts
- corn chips
- corn cereal
- oat cereal and oats
- licorice (unless you are in Norway buying Norwegian licorice)
- condiments
- caramel color
- instant coffee
- rotisserie chicken
- rice blends and mixes
- ice cream
- granola
- brewer's yeast
- sausage
- protein bars and protein cookies
- corn tortillas

- potato chips
- french fries
- salad dressing
- sauces
- marinade
- sushi
- pre-marinated or seasoned meats
- spices
- pie filling and pudding
- lunchmeat
- over the counter medications
- cosmetics
- toothpaste
- supplements
- Play-doh

Candy

Gluten is usually found in truffle candy, used as a cheap filler. The gluten-free safety of pre-packaged, store-bought candy depends on the manufacturer's season and how the candy is manufactured. Listen to Episode #63 on "Not So Scary Halloween Candy" to determine what is safe and what candy to avoid.

Malt

Malt is a sweetener which is made from barley. This liquid is pervasive in many types of foods within its various forms, including malted barley flour, malted milk, malt extract, malt syrup, malt flavoring, malt vinegar. Malt is easy to use as a sweetener and inexpensive; therefore, many companies use malt. Regular vinegar such as distilled, red wine, white wine, and apple cider are usually gluten-free and are safe to eat on a gluten-free diet. As always, read the ingredients to ensure the manufacturer didn't sneak gluten into their product via malt.

Maltodextrin

Maltodextrin can be made from corn, wheat, or potatoes. Although the FDA says this is safe for Celiac and the gluten is highly processed, my joints say otherwise. I avoid maltodextrin unless the ingredients specifically say, "Maltodextrin from corn" or "Maltodextrin from potatoes," which I know is safe.

MSG

Monosodium Glutamate, or MSG, is the additive that was widely found in Asian-American cuisine. Now taken out of many Asian dishes, you can still find MSG, used as a preservative, and to enhance flavor in many types of snack foods. Although snack foods are the most common type of food, watch out for MSG in spices, sauces, gravy mixes, and salad dressings as well. Basically, read the entire label to make sure MSG isn't in the ingredients.

Hydrolyzed Wheat

Another name for MSG, see above.

Wheatgrass

This is a plant I avoid because, even though the grass itself does not contain wheat or gluten, it is wheatgrass. Wheatgrass is grown from wheat and has a high incidence of cross-contamination. I couldn't figure out why my regular morning smoothie created pain in my legs until I made the correlation to adding a greens powder, which contained wheatgrass powder, into my smoothie. My joints would always hurt the next day. Unless you are purchasing a supplement or drink that is Certified Gluten Free, you run the risk of contaminating your body with gluten when drinking or eating any food containing wheatgrass.

Wheat Starch

Wheat Starch is wheat that has been processed to remove the presence of gluten to below 20ppm and adhere to the FDA Labeling Law. The FDA says this is safe for Celiac. I've eaten bread made with wheat starch and was in pain for the next several hours. I'd say give this one a miss as I don't trust any form of wheat in my system. If you are going to try bread or another item with wheat starch, make sure to experiment on a day where you have nothing major planned in your schedule for the next three days if your body reacts badly to wheat starch.

LISTEN TO YOUR BODY

I know people who are Celiac who react to touching gluten on a table and others who break out in hives. Yet, others who are vomiting profusely are all from gluten. If caramel color bothers you and doesn't bother someone else who has Celiac, don't eat it. Listen to what your body is telling you. Even if you have the same disease, different bodies react differently to different foods and food additives.

Like other diseases, Celiac also have a wide range of types of symptoms, and severity of symptoms. However, don't be fooled if you don't have horrible symptoms after eating gluten. If you're Celiac and eat gluten, you are damaging your small intestine to the point of no return. One of the forms of no return is Adenocarcinoma or cancer of the small intestine. My dad passed away over a decade ago. I can tell you from personal experience that this is a horrible type of cancer you definitely don't want to deal with or have!

Be safe, enjoy the right foods for your body so you can travel for many years to come!

❧ 2 ☙
GLUTEN FREE FOODS AND CERTIFIED GLUTEN FREE FOODS: WHAT'S THE DIFFERENCE?

Going shopping can be a whirlwind of confusion when you can't eat gluten. Have you seen packaging that reads "gluten-free"? You may have also seen packaging which reads "certified gluten-free." If you're new to the gluten-free world, these two labels may sound like the same type of food. However, suppose you're Celiac or have an auto-immune disease. In that case, these two labels can significantly differentiate the gluten-free quality and safety of your food.

THE MACRONUTRIENTS: GLUTEN, STARCH AND FAT

Gluten is the protein found in several different grains that were listed in Chapter 1. Other types of nutrients, called macronutrients, are starch, which equal carbohydrates, and fat. Wheat starch can be permitted as long as it has been processed to take out gluten so that the wheat starch is less than 10 parts per million and the finished product tests at 10 parts per million. The original product has to test at 10 parts per million, but the final product does. Manufacturers must use caution as the processing of foods can change the nutritional value of that food.

Personally, I have found that wheat starch still bothers me as I've tried one of these types of bread. Mistakenly, I didn't read the wrapper and assumed, since it was a brand I've used before, that it was safe. Technically, the food was safe. However, I felt like my head had been inflated with helium. My joints hurt for the transition through an international airport. Learn from my mistake - always read the wrapper, even if you've used that brand before!

WHY GLUTEN FREE FOOD ISN'T SAFE FOR CELIAC

Gluten can become airborne and can become mixed into any non-gluten food inadvertently if it is manufactured in a facility that also has wheat or other gluten-containing grains. For the gluten intolerant, gluten-free foods should be relatively safe. But for those who have a gluten allergy, or celiac disease, foods labeled "gluten free" are not a hundred percent safe.

The gluten from the factory environment, such as cross-contamination from manufacturing equipment or airborne gluten, can cross paths with gluten-free food. At this point, enough gluten can accumulate on the "gluten-free" food to add small amounts of gluten to that product. They do have some risk associated with them because they may be cross-contaminated or have high enough gluten in the product that will trigger a reaction in people with an allergy or Celiac disease.

GLUTEN FREE FOODS AND CERTIFIED GLUTEN FREE FOODS. WHAT'S THE DIFFERENCE?

Generally, gluten-free relates to food that is free from gluten. This equates to the food or product you are eating is free from gluten as an ingredient in that product. Even though the product is labeled the food may contain gluten from cross-contamination discussed earlier in this chapter.

And this is where the confusion sets in for many people. If the label says "gluten-free" on the packaging, shouldn't it be safe for me to consume?

The straight answer is "yes" and "no." Understanding labeling is one of the most critical factors in staying safe when purchasing and eating food.

Have you ever seen the symbol which contains the letters GF in bold with a bold circle around the letters with a grain of wheat and a line crossed through it? Ever wonder what the symbols stand for?

This symbol actually stands for certified gluten-free food, and this certification can come from different companies. Certified gluten-free foods can contain a minimal amount of gluten measured in parts per million. Foods that are certified gluten-free in the US have gluten levels, ranging from 20ppm to 5ppm. However, if you're Celiac, it's safe to eat them as foods under 20ppm are safe for Celiac to eat. But what about foods that read gluten-free but aren't certified? Are they safe to eat?

PRODUCTS LABELED "GLUTEN FREE"

Regular gluten-free food is generally a food free from gluten ingredients containing gluten like barley, wheat, rye, and other gluten-containing grains and products. They are labeled gluten-free, because they don't include food with gluten, but they're actually not a hundred percent safe. These foods may contain enough gluten, to create symptoms in an individual with Celiac or a gluten allergy.

Gluten can become airborne and cross-contaminate other gluten-free products in their facility. Usually, vendors will have a warning label that reads: "Produced in a facility that contains wheat." The warning may also contain information about other allergens in a facility such as peanuts, barley, shellfish, and any allergen in which consumers have had a severe allergic reaction. Although the product should be safe, we cannot assume that gluten-free food labeled "gluten-free" without certification, is not 100% safe for those of us with Celiac disease.

CERTIFIED GLUTEN-FREE FOODS: SAFE FOR CELIAC

So, what does it mean to be certified gluten-free? Certified Gluten Free means that the product is free from gluten. The product has been verified from an independent organization.

For some foods, it's hard to be 100% gluten-free. There are a few products that are simply gluten-free. For example, if you buy an apple from the store and eat it, that apple will most likely be a hundred percent gluten-free. However, pre-made packaged products are much less safe for those with Celiac disease. For ready-to-eat foods, there are several certified gluten-free food standards to ensure safety.

In August of 2017, the USA FDA delivered a directive for certified gluten-free products to be tested and confirmed with less than 20 parts per million gluten in the product. This level of gluten is determined safe for Celiac or people with gluten allergies. What does that mean?

For food, this means that in a million parts of your food product, only 20 parts contain gluten. This is a minimal amount of gluten and does not create a reaction in those of us with Celiac Disease. Even though these items may not be 100% free from gluten, foods with 20 parts per million are safe for those who have Celiac, gluten intolerance, or gluten allergy. The product has to be higher than 20 parts per million to create a reaction for those with Celiac.

Since the only treatment for Celiac disease is a strict gluten free diet, Celiac can safely eat products labeled as certified gluten free foods. So what organizations can certify foods and products as certified gluten-free?

The differences between gluten-free food and certified gluten-free foods:

Gluten Free Food	Certified Gluten Free Food
Gluten free products refer to the product as gluten free.	Certified gluten free product are certified that the products have less than 20 ppm of gluten
Not all gluten free food are safe	Certified gluten free product are 100% safe
Gluten free food are Fruit, Vegetables and Legumes, Meats, Poultry, Fish, Cereals, Grains, Breads, Biscuits, Pasta, Nuts and Cakes.	Certified gluten free food are Breads, Biscuits, Pasta, Nuts, chocolate and Cakes etc. from certified organization like "Enjoy Life Foods".

ASSOCIATIONS THAT CERTIFY GLUTEN-FREE FOOD

Currently, four associations can certify foods as gluten-free: the Gluten Intolerance Group of North America or GIG, the Gluten Free Certification Organization or GFCO, the National Celiac Association, or NCA and the Canadian Celiac Association or CCA. All of these organizations have different standards that ensure products and companies as certified gluten-free.

Like the different levels of organic certification, we see for foods like the Oregon Tilth and the California Organic Certification, the standards with certified gluten-free products also differ according to the company, which certifies the food.

There's also the Canadians Celiac Association, who require less than 20 parts per million and can certify food purchased in Canada. National Celiac Association, the strictest certification, requires less than five parts per million of gluten to receive their seal of approval.

GFCO STANDARD FOR GLUTEN FREE

If you've ever seen the capital letters "GF " in bold with a circle surrounding them, this signifies the product is Certified Gluten Free and is safe for Celiac. You can find this symbol on the front or top corner or on the back of your package next to other symbols such as Vegan or Paleo-friendly. Although a product does not have to be vegetarian to be gluten-free, some products offer both certifications.

The GF with the circle is the seal of the GFCO, Certified Gluten Free product and certifies their product is gluten-free by GFCO standards. Since GFCO standards are the conventional standard in America are the GFCO guidelines. "The GFCO mark meets both the USDA requirements as well as international trademark registration requirements."

"The Gluten Intolerance Group or GIG is an industry leader in the certification of gluten-free products and food services, announced it is rebranding the Gluten-Free Certification Organization (GFCO) mark to support its expanding presence in international markets. To date, over 60,000 products from 51 countries have earned GFCO certification. The GFCO certification program protects consumers with gluten-related disorders by confirming that a product meets strict gluten-free safety standards. GFCO companies will have until 2022 to completely adopt the new mark on the packaging."

GIG determined that a design change was required to

meet international trademark regulations to make their certification mark more easily identifiable to global consumers. "GFCO is the only gluten-free certification that holds companies and products accountable through audits, random product testing, and process surveillance. All GFCO certification bodies are accredited to ISO 17065, ensuring they follow internationally established best practices for auditing and product certification." The GFCO does not permit the use of any ingredient that consists of wheat, rye, barley, or hybrids of these grains in products certified gluten-free with the exception that care has been taken to remove the gluten.

THE QUESTIONABLE SAFETY OF OATS FOR CELIAC

Oats are another product that can be iffy because oats can be processed with farm machinery or in a factory that contains grains with gluten. There are several steps in the processing of oats that can cause cross-contamination and create unsafe food.

The process of growing, harvesting, and other creation of the oats has been approved to forestall or slow down or prevent cross-contamination. The finished product is less than 10 parts per million, it will be considered certified gluten-free. If they've been appropriately harvested and processed to be 10 parts per million or less, gasses such as wheat and barley can be certified. Also, finished products must be 10 parts per million or less. Then, any blended ingredients have to come to 10 parts per million or less. Wheat starch or oats or any ingredients you're putting together, the bottom line comes down to that finished product has to be less than 10 parts per million.

HOW TO FIND CERTIFIED GLUTEN FREE FOODS

So how can you find these safe foods to eat that are certified gluten-free? Look for the Certified Gluten Free label on packages that you buy. Check both the back and the front of the package, as there isn't an industry standard for the location of the certification logo.

Another fun way to find Certified Gluten Free foods is by searching on your favorite web browser #certifiedglutenfree. Make sure not to put spaces in the hashtag when you search! This will provide you with pages of links to sites that offer certified gluten-free food or have more information.

ONLINE RESOURCES TO FIND CERTIFIED GLUTEN FREE FOODS

The GFCO and GIG website have the buyer and distributor guide for certified gluten-free products with over 260 pages of information on certified gluten-free products. The Celiac Foundation, Canadian Celiac Foundation, and the National Celiac Foundation all have resources on their websites. Additionally, check out Chapter 5 Gluten Free Travel Apps for more information on using apps as tools to find gluten-free foods.

You can shop for certified gluten-free products by checking at stores you shop at, such as Whole Foods, Sprouts, Natural Grocers, and other natural markets. Even Walmart has a gluten-free products page, which shows all the gluten-free products Walmart carries. However, not all of these products that are listed in the gluten-free search are certified gluten-free. Definitely check out the brand's website you are going to purchase to see if they have a list of gluten-free products.

Many companies that sell gluten-free products, such as

Udis, Be Free, Schar, and Kinnikinnick, also have their own company pages, usually store locators. Find out more by searching for the company brand page online.

If you're stuck and unsure what to do, send me a message on IG @travelglutenfreepodcast or contact me through my website at www.travelglutenfreepodcast.com and I'll direct you to my favorite foods which are safe for Celiac!

❦ 3 ❧
THE CHALLENGE: EATING OUT GLUTEN-FREE

Ever heard of the phrase "food anxiety"? If you haven't and are now gluten-free, especially if you're Celiac, you will almost surely have experienced this type of stressor. Food anxiety relates to the stress caused by eating, especially when eating out. In this case, the burden is caused by being unsure if the food you have ordered or purchased, won't make you sick.

Believe me, I have had food anxiety on multiple trips and vacations. I understand how this type of nervousness can affect and even ruin a vacation. Always remember that the recommendations in this book aren't a guarantee you'll never get glutened. Even with all my experience and knowledge, I still get glutened two to three times a year. Keep in mind I travel six to eight weeks of the year and eat out about once a week. This being said, the chances of getting myself cross-contaminated are high because of the quantity of food I eat away from home.

Suppose you do follow the practices in my book. In that case, however, you will have a significantly reduced risk of becoming sick on your next vacation. Reducing the risk of accidentally eating gluten is the goal of eating out while on your journey.

TYPES OF MENUS

You may be wondering what this topic is about and why there are different "types" of menus. You may see three different types of menus listed when you read reviews for a restaurant: gluten-free menu, a labeled menu, and a dedicated menu.

Gluten-Free Menu

A gluten-free menu is a menu that a restaurant puts together that only lists gluten-free offerings. This is extremely helpful because when a server hands you a gluten-free menu, you don't have to ask what is gluten-free. Everything on that menu is gluten-free! That is a big plus when ordering because you don't have to ask the server what is OK to eat, and the server doesn't have to take time to check with the chef. Although this process is fine and I always encourage people to have the server double-check for safety. It's really nice not to have to go through this process and just choose something off a menu.

Labeled Menu

Make sure to read the key before you order from a labeled menu. A labeled menu is a menu that everyone receives but has a key to denote foods with allergen and dietary preferences such as vegetarian and vegan. Always read the key first as there isn't a consistent labeling pattern among restaurants in the US. A symbol with wheat or a G could mean either the food contains gluten, or the food is gluten-free. Usually, there will be a key at the top or bottom of the menu, which explains their food labels.

Another item you should note with a labeled menu is that sometimes a main plate or appetizer will be marked containing gluten only because this dish is served with bread. For example, many times, hummus will be labeled as containing gluten. However, it's only because this appetizer is served with naan. To date, I haven't found hummus that contains gluten in its ingredients! (That's at least one food that I know of...)

Always ask your server if the only reason the dish is labeled to have gluten is because of the bread. If they aren't sure, have them check with the chef. Remember, meats can have marinades that contain liquid gluten, so you never want to assume a dish is gluten-free.

If the dish contains gluten because of bread, ask for a substitute. You can often get apples, cucumbers, carrots, or other veggies that will nicely complement the dish without making your sick. Sometimes, you'll score big, and they will ask you if you want gluten-free bread! If not, I'm OK with a veggie or fruit substitute, and I've never been charged extra for this type of substitution.

Dedicated Gluten-Free Menu

When you are at a dedicated gluten-free restaurant, meaning the establishment doesn't serve or prepare any type of gluten in their food or in the kitchen, this is the safest place to eat. They will have a dedicated gluten-free menu. What this means for us Celiac folk is that we can eat like "normal" people and order anything we want off the menu! Dedicated restaurants are also the most likely places you'll have a choice of several different desserts to eat, besides a dedicated gluten-free bakery.

FINDING SAFE PLACES TO EAT

Finding a GF restaurant may not sound hard until you try to look for one to eat, especially in a rural area. Cities and more densely populated areas have more Celiac-friendly food choices. Every once in a while, you'll find a gluten-free friendly dining establishment in a small town. Usually, the reason is that the owner and or someone in their family is Celiac or can't eat gluten.

How does someone who is Celiac or gluten intolerant find a place to eat that is safe when you're in unfamiliar territory? You can find a guide for gluten-free restaurants in a specific city. However, in my experience, I'm never on the side of the town where these restaurants are listed.

For example, you may find a guide that lists gluten-free restaurants in New York City. New York City is densely populated. Traveling just a few miles, especially during rush hour, can easily take 30 minutes or more. If you are hungry and tired after a long day of travel, you don't want to get ready, then travel for an extended period to find a restaurant to eat at, at least I don't! Using these tools to seek out restaurants when I'm on my vacation adventure is the easiest and most efficient way to find a great gluten-free place

TELL THE RESTAURANT YOU ARE CELIAC

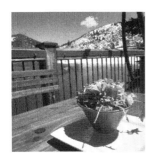

Make sure the place you are eating understands that you are eating this way because of a medical condition and not because your friend told you how she lost ten pounds because she ate a gluten-free diet! If you say you are Celiac and have a look on

their face that reflects you, you just told them you landed a spaceship nearby, explain to them you have a food allergy to gluten, not just wheat. As I have found out from experience, it's easier to tell them you have a food allergy to gluten. Many people do not understand Celiac Disease.

Dining cards are a great way to explain to your server and chef what you can and cannot eat. A great way to use dining cards is to make copies of your cards to give to the waiter or waitress at your table. Now, they can attach your card to your check so that wherever your order is sent, the people creating your meal are notified about your food limitations.

USING APPS TO FIND GLUTEN FREE DINING OPTIONS

Find Me Gluten-Free App

One of my favorite tools to find gluten-free restaurants is Find Me Gluten Free App. Jason Elmore, the creator of this app, is Celiac. He decided to make the app after being frustrated about the difficulty of finding food that is safe to eat at restaurants.

To find out more about Jason and how he created the Find Me Gluten Free App, check out Episode #10 of the Travel Gluten Free Podcast!

The basic version of the app is free. Celiac and gluten-intolerant individuals can use the app to find safe food all over the world. Each restaurant has user ratings and reviews, which is extremely helpful when looking for a place to eat. When considering reviews, consider how long ago the review was written and if they are writing a fair review.

The search option gives you the ability to put in a city, zip code, name of a location, or both! You can also search by ethnic cuisine, which is one of the features I love because I can search for the type of dish, I'm in the mood to eat.

The local icon at the bottom of the app gives you many options, such as:

- Most Celiac friendly
- Dedicated gluten free
- Open now (which is great when you are traveling in Utah because many places are closed on Sundays)
- My bookmarks
- Best rated
- Closest
- By address or city
- Takeout
- Delivery
- By category
- Lunch
- Chains

You'll want to remember what restaurants you ate so you can tell your friends or write about your new discovery on social media. Bookmark the restaurant. All the places you bookmark will show under your account! If you can't remember where the restaurant was because you stopped at several towns, you can easily click the map of the restaurant to see its location.

You can see the most recent gluten-free reviews for each restaurant by clicking on the Activity icon at the bottom of the app. A list of reviews, starting with the most current, are listed so you can find new and most recently updated reviews.

This app has excellent features in the free version; however, if you take road trips or travel frequently, I'd definitely suggest making the investment and purchasing the paid version. The upgraded app features many of the filters listed above, such as 'open now' and tells you the restaurant's geographical direction. This feature saves you time when you are traveling on the road to find places to eat in the direction that you are going.

Features include: Search Near Me, Search by Name, Recent Activity, and my favorite, the Dining Card.

What is the Dining Card? Do you ever get tired of explaining to people that bread has gluten? Do you believe that most people who don't eat gluten live in a cave all day and refuse information about food and nutrition? The Dining Card must have been created with the less-than- knowledgeable server in mind! It starts off with "Hi, I have Celiac Disease/ severe gluten intolerance" and explains in one easy paragraph what you cannot eat. It also highlights specific grains you cannot eat and some common yet not-so-obvious foods (such as oyster sauce), which contain gluten.

100% Gluten-Free App

Trying to find dedicated gluten-free restaurants on your travel adventure? This app is going to be a great travel assistant. The only app that lists 100% dedicated gluten-free restaurants will be able to find gluten-free bakeries, restaurants, food trucks, breweries, and more with the click of a button. Listing only restaurants that are dedicated gluten-free, every place to eat on this app is safe for Celiac!

When you open the app, it automatically filters places to eat by location closest to you. When you see a location, you can also see the category or type of eatery this establishment is listed under. This makes it simple to find the kind of food you're in the mood to eat. You can also search and or filter by type of eatery, such as

- Bakery
- Cafe

- Brewery
- Catering
- Food truck
- Grocery store
- Ice cream / gelato (the most important category for myself!)
- Restaurant

You can also search by distance, how many miles away you are willing, or not willing to travel. Expanding your search can also be a good option if you do not find a good selection of safe places to eat.

This app is free to use, and if you come across a new place to eat that is not listed on the app, you can add that location so others that are gluten-free will be able to find and eat at that location!

USING ONLINE SEARCH TOOLS TO FIND GLUTEN-FREE DINING

OpenTable

An online resource I love to use when booking a table is 'Opentable.' This site is an online reservation site, which also has an app version. You can find them on the web at opentable.com. You can use OpenTable, or use their mobile app, 'Opentable,' to find and make reservations. In return for using their service, you receive points once you've dined at that restaurant. When you reach a certain amount of points, you can receive dining rewards through Opentable.

If you're going to make a reservation, you might get points and take advantage of rewards through Opentable. Sign up for a free account and search for where you went to eat. You can choose how many people are dining, the date you want to eat out, and the time you want. Your other available filters are location, restaurant or type of cuisine, including gluten-free! You also have the choice of checking gluten-free and another kind of cuisine, such as vegetarian, vegan, Indian, Italian, or whatever type of food you are craving.

On the "Neighborhood" filter is where you can filter by cuisine. Suppose I'm in the mood for Italian. In that case, I can check Italian. If I want to look at Italian, Spanish, and Vegetarian, I can check off all three. Other filters on this site are Meat, Asian, Continental, Dim Sum, European, Mediterranean, Middle Eastern, Wine bar, and many other choices. My three favorite filters when looking for restaurants are Gluten-free, 'Top Rated,' and 'Romantic.'

Opentable does not have every time slot that is available at that location. If you don't see the time you want at the restaurant you want to eat, you can call the restaurant and reserve directly with them, although you won't get points. If you're trying to reserve and the website says that there's only one-time slot left. You definitely want that restaurant, but at a different time, call and double-check with the restaurant to see if they have other times available that are not listed on Opentable.

You can read customer reviews on Opentable as well. For example, one restaurant I really love in Park City is The Mustang. Opentable reads, "Rating of four and a half out of five stars. It has 612 ratings, and 88 people recommend The Mustang". This restaurant is listed as "Contemporary American." I can see quite a bit of information about that restaurant.

When sorting your search results, you can sort them by featured, A to Z, by highest rated, and price. When I search ratings and sort by highest rated restaurant based on my search parameters, Fireside Dining, Deer Valley Resort came up the highest with 94 percent recommended and the best overall rating. Firewood came up with 'Fit for Foodies', and 97 percent recommended, Shabu came up with 'Exceptional,' and 94 percent recommended.

Restaurants can also be filtered by price with $, $$, $$$, $$$$. $$ sign is $30 and the $$$ sign, which is $31 to $50 per entree and $$$$, which is $50 and over per entree. Now keep in mind that sometimes these aren't exactly sorted correctly because one time I went to a restaurant 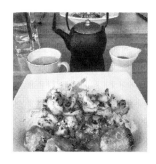 that had a $$ sign price and it was definitely a $$$ price. You can always double-check their menu online for entree pricing to see if it fits within your budget.

TripAdvisor

When you think of this website, you usually think of traveling. Still, TripAdvisor is a great way to find local food in your town, especially if you live in an area that benefits tourism.

Go to TripAdvisor and set up a free account. Look up your local town or the town you are going to visit. When I look up restaurants in Park City, where I live, I can browse by food or community picks. If I browse by a 'Community Pick,' I can see that others on the site feature foods and restaurants they like.

They have online reservations, cuisines, and dishes as options to search under and filter. So, if I look under 'Cuisines and Dishes,' I can find lots of different ethnic choices that they have on here, like the Caribbean, Barbecue, Spanish, Southwestern, and the Mediterranean. Norwegian. Having the cuisine listed on the sidebar does not denote that cuisine is served in the city you are searching in. The cuisine options list all cuisines around the world that are represented on TripAdvisor. They also have gluten-free options under the 'Dietary Restriction' category.

They also have vegetarian-friendly, vegan options, and Kosher. If I click on 'gluten-free,' I can see the list of restaurants in Park City with my filters on TripAdvisor for restaurants that offer gluten-free options. Results are Five5eeds, River Horse on Main, Seven 710 Bodega, Harvest, 501 on Main. Powder, Handle, Twisted Fern, and a variety of other restaurants came up under the gluten-free options checkmark.

You can further filter restaurants by checking off more categories such as 'Romantic' and applying them. Cross-reference your restaurant(s) you have found with, 'Find Me Gluten Free or 100% Gluten Free app. Again, always double-check by calling and asking the 'Three Questions' of the restaurant.

Use #hashtags to find gluten-free foods

I've found amazing places to eat, including bakeries, while using hashtags to find gluten-free food! I will tell you that this definitely works better in more substantial metropolitan areas than smaller, less populated ones. For example, if I looked up #glutenfreeParkCity, I would see very few posts. However, if I looked up #glutenfreeutah, I would see more posts, except that Utah is a vast state, and the post from which this was tagged could easily be a three-hour drive from my location.

If you are in a city or largely populated area, look for the hashtag and the city you are visiting. When I visited London, I looked up #glutenfreelondon. I found a dedicated gluten-free bakery two miles away from where I was staying. Unfortunately, I wasn't able to get there as the restaurant we chose to eat at, which I also found under the same hashtag, was in the opposite direction of the bakery. Additionally, the bakery closed in the early afternoon, and we had just unpacked from our long, overseas flight. I was simply too tired to make the trip to the bakery that day.

I'm definitely going to make that bakery the next time I'm in London!

If the state you are in is small, like New Hampshire, you can use the hashtag #glutenfreenewhampshire, and you're able to find places to eat within a shorter driving distance. Use #glutenfree (add the name of the city or state here) or search using regional names if the region you are in is bigger than a small town.

Additionally, you can also use #(airportyouarein) to find out what is going on at the airport. You have a layover at or are waiting for a plane. This can be an excellent way to plan ahead of time if you are going to an airport you haven't yet!

Lastly, you can search on Google, Pinterest, or other search engines for #glutenfree (city or state). You will find any post from a blog, social media platform, or website that is tagged with the hashtag you are searching for. You may have to look through more information. However, you may also find an exciting place to eat that wasn't posted on Instagram.

LOOK for a Local Gluten-Free Blogger

Find a local, gluten-free blogger, influencer, blogger, or IG individual to view their restaurant suggestions. Let them know you are coming to their town and where you are staying and ask them for advice on their favorite dining digs. They are usually happy to share great insights into their favorite local dining spots.

CROSS-CHECKING AND REFERENCING GLUTEN-FREE DINING OPTIONS FOR ACCURACY

Now, if you want to cross-check restaurants, there are a few different options. You can ask somebody who has dined at that restaurant before. You can cross-check your results with the 'Find Me Gluten Free app or 100% Gluten-Free App. Search for the restaurant's hashtag or handle on Instagram or Pinterest to see what others are writing and posting about the place you are looking at to eat. Additionally, you should always call or visit the restaurant directly to get a feel for the safety and service of their gluten-free offerings.

CALL AND CONTACT the Restaurant Directly

Even if the restaurant has rave reviews, call the restaurant or bakery to verify that they're gluten-free. Don't ruin your vacation by getting sick from eating cross-contaminated food or getting accidentally "glutened" if someone serves the wrong food.

ASK the Right Questions

First, you want to ask the eating establishment if they offer gluten-free items on their menu. If the person you're talking to is not sure, ask them if they are new to the restaurant. If they aren't, this could be a red flag. If they are a recent hire, ask to talk to another member of the wait staff, the Maître d' or the chef.

Ask them point-blank, "What choices do you offer for gluten-free? So do you offer anything besides salads?". Sometimes a dining establishment will only offer salads as "gluten-free choices," which is OK if you're in the mood for a salad.

More often than not, especially for dinner, I'd like a more substantial meal.

They should tell you which menu items are gluten-free and which selections can be made gluten-free so you can get an idea of what food choices you have from that restaurant. If you have asked two or three people in the restaurant, or no one sounds confident in telling you food choices, this is a sure sign that this establishment is not gluten-free friendly. Do not go to that restaurant to eat.

Next, ask them "How do you prep gluten-free food?", "Do you have a separate kitchen area for gluten-free?", "Do you wipe everything down for Celiacs?" If the person on the other end of the line can confidently answer your question and understands or can explain their procedure for allergy-safe preparation, then you can pretty much bet that that's a safe place to eat.

Never Accept the Phrase "I'm pretty sure" for an Answer

When you ask any staff a question and respond with the phrase "I'm pretty sure" for an answer, do not accept that answer. If they tell you they're 'pretty sure,' it's safe, and they're not giving you anyone else to talk to, or they're not taking down your number to have somebody call you back. Skip that restaurant. This is a huge red flag that this establishment does not have a gluten-free protocol, and if they do, they haven't trained their staff in the safety of providing gluten-free food.

When someone has this phrase in their answer to me, I always respond with, "Would you please check with the chef because if I eat gluten, I will be sick for days." This gives them a good idea that you are not eating gluten-free for your fad diet and that your health is essential. After replying with this phrase, my server will go back and check with the chef

99% of the time. When they come back with your answer, double-check by asking, "You checked with the chef, and they said, (repeat their answer)." If they didn't check with the chef, you would be able to see their eyes shift or look away. If your server doesn't want to make an effort, then talk with the maître' D' to have a different waiter or leave the restaurant immediately. I would never risk my health with wait staff that won't go the extra mile.

Be Bold When Asking for Your Health and Safety

Definitely, don't be shy about asking questions and confirming answers with the wait staff. I'm always asking questions about food, and if my server or the staff are upset because I have to put my health first, then that's obviously not a place that I feel safe eating. I'm not going to go there. This equates to the people that I eat with are not going to eat there, and that also means that I'm not going to frequent that restaurant in the future.

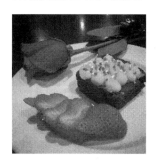

Another thing you might want to do, too, is what we did on Valentine's Day, is we brought our own bread so that I had bread to eat. So, ask them, "Can I bring in my own dessert and bread?". We went to a gluten free bakery in Salt Lake, 'Sweet Cakes Bakery' and got their squash roles which are super delicious and gluten-free brownies to bring with us for dinner.

We brought our gluten-free items with us to dinner. The wait staff served the gluten-free bread and dessert with the regular bread, and my husband got a regular dessert. They served me the brownie with some ice cream, which was really great.

Ask the restaurant if you can bring in your own gluten-free bread and dessert if they do not offer these menu selections because you are Celiac. Usually, they'll be pretty accommodating. If they aren't accommodating, try a different restaurant.

Insist on Your Choice of Restaurant

Do you really need to be selfish when it comes to eating out? YES, if you have limited choices because of your dietary restrictions. Your health must come first! Feeling bad because you think others are losing out? Drop that feeling of guilt because that other person wouldn't feel the same about the situation if they were in your shoes.

People who aren't gluten-free don't understand what we go through, they think it's silly or our digestive discomfort isn't that bad, and we should just put up with it. Seriously? When is the last time anyone enjoyed having pain and stomach cramps for three days because they ate a doughnut? Maybe some twisted masochist, but for the rest of us who want to live and eat, we would instead feel good and eat good food, just like everyone else.

Take that gluten-free app, your restaurant guide, or your friend's advice and insist you eat at the restaurant you CAN eat. The person that says, "Well, hey, they have salads!" tell them the last time you checked, you found out you were not a manatee.

Be Proactive and Speak Up!

When you go out to eat, be proactive about choosing a restaurant that offers gluten-free options and follows precautions against cross-contamination. Use the tips and tools found in this guide to select a restaurant that can accommodate your needs. A bit of research may be required. However, you will be glad you spent the time when you are eating at a new restaurant without worry.

Talk to your server and to the manager about how to avoid cross-contamination. Ask your server to check with the chef about the safety of menu items, and confirm your food is gluten-free when it arrives. Tell your server you have an allergy (even though we really know we don't have an allergy, but we need to speak to the unknowing sometimes). Tell them that eating gluten-free is not a choice, you will be extremely sick if you eat gluten. Make sure to say 'extremely' before 'sick.' I noticed this ups the level of concern with your server to get your food order correct.

Walk Out If You Feel Unsafe

If your server is not concerned, has no idea what to do, or at any time you don't feel safe eating at a restaurant, just walk out. It's not worth the risk of getting sick, especially when you are traveling. Don't worry about the feelings of the people at the restaurant. When the servers and staff of the establishment aren't concerned about your health, that is not a place you need to be.

I've walked out of places after sitting down to eat when I've talked to the server, and they were clueless. I respectfully said, "Thank You, but I don't believe I can eat safely" and excused myself. I went on to find a different establishment where I could eat without experiencing food anxiety. Isn't that the whole point of a vacation is to be relaxed and worry-free?

Be your best gluten-free self! Be bold, fearless, and insist on your choice of eating establishment. Your health is just as

THE GUIDE TO TRAVELING GLUTEN FREE

important as the other people in your dining party. Because, after all, your taste buds need to be satisfied just like everyone else!

You should be able to find gluten-free on your journey. It's sometimes tricky, but when you keep looking, there's usually a gem amid the dust and sand of gluten-laden places to eat!

You can find amazing gluten-free food when you know the right tools to use!

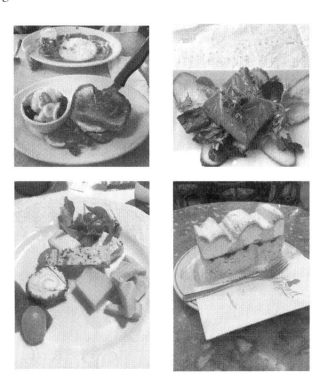

❦ 4 ❦

HOW TO PLAN AHEAD AND BE READY FOR GLUTEN FREE TRAVEL

Planning a vacation in and of itself can be a daunting task - especially if you have little ones in your party. Throw celiac disease, gluten intolerance, or a food allergy on board. Now you feel like you want to jump off that cruise bow into the water like Rose in the movie Titanic.

However, I'm here to tell you that traveling gluten-free, although having its challenges, can be done with the right tools, planning, and a bit more time and patience. No matter what type of travel you choose—boat, car, plane, train, or cruise—the best advice I can give you is to be prepared. Make sure you know what to do ahead of time, and always call the place where you booked your travel plans to find out the specifics.

When I first started traveling without the ability to eat gluten, I thought, "Wow, this is going to be freaking challenging." I know from my own first-hand experience how challenging it can be to travel gluten free. You'll need to think ahead and plan, with a little more work and preparation, you should feel safe and ready to enjoy your vacation!

DOWNLOAD APPS AHEAD OF TIME

I have several suggestions for apps you can use when you are traveling. Download these apps ahead of time. If they have an option to use the app without Wi-Fi, definitely use that option. When you are a gluten-free traveler, having a cell phone with a substantial amount of storage is a necessity—not a choice. Between downloading useful apps and taking photos of your food, you will need a cell phone with a decent amount of storage. See Chapter 5, Gluten Free Travel Apps for information on apps you can use for easier gluten-free travel.

PRINT PAPER MAPS

Even if you have data, you can't always get a good connection when you are traveling. If there are restaurants you want to go to, especially if you are going to a country where you don't speak the language, I recommend printing up a map with the location of the place you would like to dine. You can easily find a local to give you directions when you can show them a physical map. Additionally, you don't have to worry about handing over your phone to a stranger who could run off with your device!

You can also purchase local city maps online for many different cities worldwide. Marking or making a key with the places you would like to eat is an easy way to see where these dining options are located when you are out and about your adventure. Easily pack these in your travel bag and keep them with you wherever you go.

CARRYING GLUTEN FREE FOOD

Even though travel is definitely a bit harder with celiac disease, you can have a safe and fun-filled trip with a bit of diligence on your part. Make sure to cover your bases before you go on your journey. This said, your most intricate and detailed plans can be derailed, which is why I always carry food with me no matter where I'm going. I'd rather carry around some extra food then be stuck without anything to eat when traveling.

Use a backpack, large shoulder bag, or other bags that are roomy enough to keep your essentials plus some food. I'd also recommend taking a metal water bottle with you as plastic bottles can break more easily than metal. Additionally, I find metal bottles easier to keep clean than plastic, which can be porous and hold tannins from your iced or cold tea and residual flavor from previous drinks.

PACKING YOUR LUGGAGE AND CARRY-ON

This is the biggest challenge when traveling gluten-free. Depending on their mood and the amount of sleep the TSA agent had, you may get someone who is sympathetic or an agent who is gleefully pulling the entire contents out of your bag.

TSA has limits to the amount of a single liquid you can take on

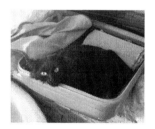

Although your cat is not considered a "liquid," you don't want to pack him in your carry-on!

your carry-on. Find out more details on their website. You can also use the TSA checklist to review what to do before you fly. Find more detail on packing your bags for flying in Chapter 11 How to Pack Your Travel Bags. Find out what you

should pack, what you shouldn't pack, and the current TSA rules and
resources.

LEAVE ROOM IN YOUR LUGGAGE FOR "SOUVENIR FOOD"

When I go on a vacation, I bring back food every time. I'm definitely an exotic salt lover, so my cabinet has almost a dozen different types of salt. I bring many of them back as "souvenirs" of my trip. Check out my IG post on the licorice salt I brought back from Iceland!

Additionally, I'm always game for a yummy gluten-free dessert or bring back a gluten-free food I've not found anywhere else. While you most likely have packed food for your trip that would have been eaten and have left some space, make sure to leave extra room in your luggage as you will most likely find a gluten-free goodie to take home with you!

You can buy a collapsible duffle or travel bag that is flat and takes up very little space. When you are ready to go home, you can unfold the bag, pack it full of goodies, and bring your delectable finds back with you.

THE EASIEST GLUTEN FREE TRIP

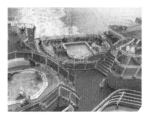

If you want to take a trip with the least amount of preparation when food is involved, I would highly recommend a cruise. I was so against cruising when I first started traveling on my own because I felt I wouldn't experience local culture on a deeper level. While that is true to some extent, what you don't have to worry about is having safe food. When you're Celiac or can't eat gluten because of health reasons, this benefit outweighs the loss of being able to make your own schedule.

Cruises are a fantastic way to enjoy a place without the worry of being cross-contaminated. Why? Cruises are incredibly service-oriented, especially when it comes to dining. I have never talked to anyone who has been sick on a cruise because they have been glutened. Check out my podcast Episodes #39 and #40 and Chapter 15 on Cruising Gluten Free to find out more.

THE MOST CHALLENGING GLUTEN FREE TRIP

Train rides would be the hardest to eat safely, as they do not have room for a separate kitchen. Train kitchens are small because of space limitations. If you are a sensitive celiac, I would advise you not to eat the food on a multi-day train ride. When traveling by train, plan ahead to bring food on board to eat. Another option is to eat when you stop at cities on your itinerary to have a safer food experience.

ALWAYS CALL AHEAD TO CONFIRM

Whether you are traveling by train, boat, cruise line, or airplane, always call ahead to confirm the company you are going with knows your dietary limitations. I suggest calling 30 days ahead of time, as many businesses require you to call well in advance of your trip. If you're traveling on the last-minute deal or booking less than 30 days in advance, telephone to ensure you can still get safe food if your ticket price involves meals. NEVER ASSUME they will have safe food for you to eat!

Whichever way you choose to travel, be sure to do your

research and plan ahead! If you ever have questions about planning for your trip, I'd be glad to assist you. Reach out to me on my contact form at www.travelglutenfreepodcast.com/contact-us.html

If your server is not concerned, has no idea what to do, or at any time you don't feel safe eating at a restaurant, just walk out. It's not worth the risk of getting sick, especially when you are traveling. Don't worry about the feelings of the people at the restaurant. When the servers and staff of the establishment aren't concerned about your health, that is not a place you need to be.

I've walked out of places after sitting down to eat when I've talked to the server, and they were clueless. I respectfully said, "Thank You, but I don't believe I can eat safely" and excused myself. I went on to find a different establishment where I could eat without experiencing food anxiety. Isn't that the whole point of a vacation is to be relaxed and worry-free?

Be your best gluten-free self! Be bold, fearless, and insist on your choice of eating establishment. Your health is just as important as the other people in your dining party. Because, after all, your taste buds need to be satisfied just like everyone else!

5
USING GLUTEN FREE APPS TO SHOP FOR SAFE FOOD

Have you been searching the internet to plan where you are going to eat for your next travel adventure only to be frustrated after hours of searching? Google can be a great resource. However, when you want to efficiently search for safe, gluten-free food, the best avenue is by downloading and using gluten-free apps. Navigate your gluten-free world quickly and effectively using these tools.

With these apps, you'll have an easier time of being and finding gluten-free food, several different apps are fantastic resources to find a gluten-free diet. Some of the following app options are available online, as well.

Find Me Gluten Free App

Check out a description of this app in Chapter 3, where I talk about how to find safe restaurants when you travel.

100% Gluten Free App

Created by Carrie from For Gluten Sake, this app features

restaurants that are dedicated gluten-free only! No worrying about cross-contamination when you eat at these locations, 100% Gluten Free App is an excellent resource for finding restaurants to eat at sans gluten. Read more about this app in Chapter 3, where I talk about how to find safe restaurants.

Eat! GF

This app has some really cool features, including lists of companies, products, services, and recipes. You can also create an account with the app and store your favorite foods on your list with your account. Find certified gluten-free products by the company or search in the app for products that are certified gluten-free.

Celiac Disease Foundation app also contains resources from the Celiac Disease Foundation website. Find items such as meal plans, healthcare providers, directory, and symptoms checklist, at www.Celiac.org.

GF Scanner

GF Scanner allows you to scan the barcode on a product. After scanning the bar code, this app will tell you if the product is gluten-free. I don't know if that app will tell you if it's certified gluten-free, but it will tell you if it is a gluten-free product, you can always cross-check that with the company website.

Makeena

If you have to be gluten-free, you might as well make money! Makeena is a fantastic tool where you can discover new gluten-free brands and find your favorites. Download the Makeena app, create a free account, search for brands you love, and get back cash rebates on the food you already buy, including organic produce!

Search for products under categories. Once you've found a product you are going to purchase, read the description for the rebate. Usually, you'll have to take a picture of your receipt and/or the product barcode as proof of purchase. Next, rack up your rebate $$$ and earn points on the app which you can redeem for free items!

It's super easy to use. Check out the "How to Redeem" section for simple, step-by-step instructions on how to utilize this fantastic money-saving app!

Schar Gluten Free

Next, one of my favorite companies, which makes such gluten-free goodies, is Schar. Their app gives you information on their gluten-free products, a list of the product's characteristics such as preservative-free, palm oil-free, nutritional information, and a picture of the product. In the app, you'll also find a list of stores that carry their products.

My favorite feature in this app? Schar also provides a travel option that will show you a list of stores within a designated radius of your location that carries Schar gluten-free. If I am at home, it will show me stores in my current position. However, if I'm traveling, say I'm in San Diego. I can take the location slider and create a search up to 125 miles around me. The app will show all the locations within that radius with Schar gluten-free products, which is a really great feature.

And as you know, part of my podcast talks about travel. So that is a great feature to have on an app if you are traveling and gluten-free, and you're looking to buy some really yummy Schar goodies. And of course, what great food app wouldn't have recipes? Of course, Schar has recipes as well!

. . .

Is That Gluten Free?

Another app, Is That Gluten Free, is 7.99, so it is slightly on the pricey side. Look for brands and search products, and if the product has a green checkmark, it is safe and gluten-free.

❧ 6 ☙
STORES THAT OFFER GLUTEN FREE FOODS

When shopping on vacation, I highly recommend purchasing as many Certified Gluten Free products and foods sourced from dedicated gluten-free companies. Spending the extra money on safe food when you travel and having a great adventure is absolutely worth the additional 10 to 20% more you will spend on food. See Chapter 2 to discover why Certified Gluten Free is the only 100% safe choice for Celiacs.

Each store has a sample listing of gluten-free products. However, this list is only a small quantity of gluten-free foods each market has available in store. Shopping online can yield a wider variety of gluten-free choices that can be shipped to your travel location ahead of time! Remember that not all stores carry the same food products, so always check for availability online or while shopping.

WALMART

If you're looking to save money on your gluten-free budget, shopping at Walmart is a great way to bring down your grocery bill. Walmart actually has a large selection of gluten-free products in their grocery section in the gluten-free aisle. Walmart offers many popular gluten-free brands such as Schar, Udi's, Kinnikinnick, and its signature Great Value brand gluten-free products.

In addition to their dedicated gluten-free section, you can also find gluten-free food throughout the store in produce, frozen, and non-refrigerated aisles. Find a comprehensive list of Walmart's gluten-free products on their website https://bit.ly/39uiwtV

Popular Gluten Free Products at Walmart

Caulipower pizza
Udi's gluten-free pizza
Amy's gluten-free frozen burrito
Livekuna quinoa flour
Nature's Eats blanched almond flour
Better Body organic coconut flour.
Purely Elizabeth gluten-free granola
Superfood Granola
Van's gluten-free cereal
Great Value gluten-free pancake and waffle mix
King Arthur gluten-free pie crust mix
Schar Schnack Cakes and bread rolls
Gluten Freeda oatmeal
Great Value gluten-free sandwich cookies

TARGET

Target has always been a fun place to grocery shop as it carries its own brand line and other popular healthy brands at great prices. According to Target, their brand is defined by their "Good and Gather" concept that is quality food made without artificial synthetic colors, artificial sweeteners. Find a comprehensive list of their gluten-free foods here https://bit.ly/39vNKR2

Popular Gluten Free Product Brands Found at Target

Banza Chickpea Rice
Uncle Ben's Boil-in-Bag White Rice
Hinode Calrose Medium Grain Rice
RiceSelect Royal Rice Blend
WOW Baking Company Chocolate Chip Cookies
Quest Tortilla Style Protein Chips
EPIC Chili Lime Pork Rinds
EPIC Bison Uncured Bacon & Cranberry Nutrition Bar
Cheetos Crunchy Flamin Hot - 8.5oz

COSTCO

As you may have found out, gluten-free food costs more than non-gluten-free foods. Why? Non-gluten free grains aren't made in the large quantities that wheat and other gluten-containing grains are created. Since their volume is lower, they cost more, hence supply and demand pricing. Luckily, Costco offers the option of buying gluten-free products in bulk, which saves us money!

Costco has a great selection of gluten-free products such as flours, spices, pasta, produce, and foods in every shopping category. They also offer gluten-free products in their own brand line of food, Kirkland. Offering gluten free selections at affordable pricing, this is a win for those of us who are gluten free. Find a complete list of gluten-free foods here https://bit.ly/2CQZpyb

Product Brands Costco Carries

Beanitos Chips
Gratify Pretzel Thins
Aidels meatballs and sausage
Beyond Meat veggie burgers

Kirkland Roasted Turkey Deli Meat
CoCo-Roons
Harvest Stone gluten free crackers
Mary's Crackers
Kirkland Seaweed

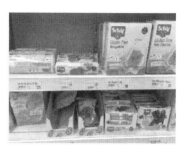

Schar is a brand that is carried all over the world! I found this stash of Schar in Austria.

SAFEWAY

Safeway has a large variety of food that is safe for Celiac. This market chain prides itself on offering a wide range of gluten-free bakery products, including a delicious assortment of gluten-free bread, doughnuts, and cookies. You can easily find gluten-free food items throughout the store, as these foods are highlighted with a unique gluten-free tag! Find a complete list of gluten-free choices here https://bit.ly/32TKFJn

GLUTEN FREE FOODS OFFERED AT SAFEWAY

Ener-G Foods Inc
Glutino
Kinnikinnick
The Olson's Baking Co.
UDI's

KROGER

Shopping at Kroger stores, such as Smith's Grocery Store, will give you a large variety of gluten-free and dairy-free foods. In addition to providing many different gluten-free foods, Smith's also has a clearance section in the back of the store where you can find gluten-free loaves of bread, baked goods, and other foods for under $2! To save even more, make sure to download the store app, open a free account, and "clip" digital coupons for your favorite gluten-free foods.

While you can find gluten-free throughout the store, check out their natural and organic food aisles. They also carry gluten-free foods in their store brand, Simple Truth, an organic food brand. Find more great gluten-free items on their website at https://bit.ly/2D4VaPd

<u>Gluten Free Food Choices at Kroger Stores</u>
Udi's bread
Kite Hill non-dairy yogurt
Oatly oat milk
Snack Factory Gluten Free Pretzel Crisps
Skinny Pop Popcorn
Kettle Honey Dijon Chips
Quaker gluten free oats
Simple Mills crackers
Envirokidz cereals
Van's gluten free waffles

WHOLE FOODS

Whole Foods also carries an extensive list of vegan, paleo, and keto-friendly brands in addition to many gluten-free items. Check out their website for food guides, grocery lists, meal plans, and shopping tips. Download the Amazon app, click on the Whole Foods tab and scan the QR code at checkout to receive exclusive in-store savings for Amazon Prime Members. Find out more gluten-free food choices at https://bit.ly/2EcGaiK

<u>Whole Foods Popular Gluten Free Products</u>
Noosa Coconut Yogurt
Lundberg Farms BBQ Rice Chips
Blue Diamond Pecan Nut Thins
Tate's Gluten Free Chocolate Chip Cookies
Pamela's Products Honey Grahams
Erewhon Organic Crispy Brown Rice Cereal
Alter Eco Rainbow Quinoa
BioNaturae Gluten Free Elbows
Jovial Egg Tagliatelle
KaPop! Ancient grain snacks

LOCAL HEALTH FOOD STORES

While big supermarkets and stores are great to shop at, especially if you are on vacation, seek local health food stores! Easily find local stores by searching on a map app on your mobile device. Usually, a search under the term "health food store" will render a significant list of local stores that carry a variety of gluten-free items.

When I was in New Smyrna last year, I came across a local health food store that I had passed many times when I lived in Florida. Heath's Natural Foods was a mecca of gluten-free food choices, some of which I had never seen in my local grocery stores! One of the associates asked me if I needed assistance, I told her I was Celiac and looking for gluten-free food. She showed me several options, one of which was Katz cupcakes in the refrigerated section! I bought an entire box, even though I was leaving the next day. Luckily, my daughter Aliyah, who is also Celiac, was a team player and assisted me in eating them! Since they were individually wrapped, we could take two of them in our carry-on bag for the flight home.

The benefit of going to a local health food store instead of a large chain market is the associate's level of knowledge. Many local stores hire folks who have a background in healthy eating, living, and experience. They can show you their favorite types of foods, recommend different teas and herbs, and send you home with the latest delectable gluten-free dessert!

Unfortunately, you are unlikely to find health food stores in towns with small populations. Rural towns may not even have a supermarket, let alone a health food store. Plan ahead to see the variety of health food stores in the area you will be vacationing. This will give you a good idea of how easily accessible gluten-free food is where you'll be staying.

RURAL SUPERMARKETS

Take a look in and see what gluten-free offerings smaller food markets have, you may be surprised to find a selection of gluten-free foods. When you find rural supermarkets with gluten-free food, usually the owner or manager, or someone in their immediate family, is gluten-free. They may carry bread, pasta, and some gluten-free basics in their store. Don't immediately discount rural supermarkets! Take a quick spin to see if they have safe food to offer and support a local family-owned business.

7

HOW TO AVOID GLUTEN WHILE TRAVELING

If you've had Celiac disease for a while, you already know how to avoid gluten. Removing gluten from your everyday life can be a challenging and exhausting task. Remember to watch out for sneaky gluten as well. This type of gluten is usually the variety that will make people sick.

So, what should you do to avoid another accidental ingestion in the future? Here are some simple steps to start implementing now, if you haven't already.

ALL GLUTEN-FREE FOOD IS NOT CREATED THE SAME

Your favorite pre-packaged snack in the United States or Canada may not have the same ingredients in Germany or Mexico. When traveling internationally, NEVER assume the ingredients are the same in different countries. Unless the packaged item you are eating is from a company that creates EXCLUSIVELY gluten-free foods, don't trust that the ingredients are the same. I've seen corn chips from the same manufacturer in America with the same type of labeling. The only difference was the shape of the corn chip. Guess what? One had gluten, and the other chip didn't contain gluten! Always read the ingredients regardless of the brand.

LOOK FOR CERTIFIED GLUTEN-FREE

Always check food labels. First, look for the label "Certified Gluten Free." Gluten-Free Certification labels differ according to the country you are visiting. If you are unsure, ask the staff at a health food store for assistance.

When traveling, I will gladly pay a premium for certified gluten-free food. That $2 to $3 I've paid above and beyond the other non-certified food is like buying trip insurance. If the food is certified gluten-free, then I know as a Celiac, that it's safe for me to eat. I'd rather go down that road than spend my vacation in bed rather than enjoying my adventure.

KEEP GLUTEN OUT OF YOUR VACATION KITCHEN

When traveling, keep a gluten-free kitchen if possible. You may need to use separate utensils and cookware to avoid cross-contamination. Additionally, you can use the utensils first before others who are preparing food with gluten. Ask your travel companions to eat gluten-free at your vacation place the entire week to avoid cross-contamination, especially if you are using a shared kitchen when you are on vacation.

LABEL FOOD PACKAGES WHICH EVERYONE HAS ACCESS TOO

If some of your family members don't follow a gluten-free diet, make sure everything is labeled, so you know what you can and cannot eat. Items such as toasters, cutting boards, pots/pans, and other kitchen utensils need to be kept separate or cleaned thoroughly at all times. Make sure to clean cookware and utensils immediately after eating to reduce the risk of cross-contamination.

An easy way to do this is to purchase neon stickers, such as the stickers used for pricing items at yard sales. Pick a color to represent gluten-free food and put that color sticker on all packages gluten-free to quickly identify the food. I use neon green to identify gluten-free food in my household, which is easily seen against the various food packaging. This makes it especially easy for little ones who are gluten-free to find foods they can eat without hassle.

AVOID CROSS-CONTAMINATION

Non-Celiac folks do not understand how little gluten we need to have in our system to have a severe reaction. I explain it to non-gluten-free people like this, "Yes, I could eat that piece of (fill-in-the-blank), but in 15 minutes, I'll start to feel sick. And as long as you want to hold my hair while I puke for the next six hours straight and then take care of me for the next two days, I'll eat that (fill-in-the-blank).

The last time I had to pull out my speech, I was at a business networking holiday event. One of the people in my business network group was like, oh, just eat one piece of the pie. I explicitly pointed to the bathroom of the clubhouse across the hall when I gave him my gluten-free speech, also adding I didn't think the clubhouse would be open until 3am.

Unless everyone else in your party is gluten-free or traveling alone, you'll need to take steps to avoid cross-contamination. Thoroughly and carefully cleaning your dinnerware, especially when camping, is one of the essential steps to prevent cross-contamination. You can avoid cross-contamination to clean your own silverware and put your set in a glass on a counter or in a separate storage bin. Labeling your gluten-free silverware, plates, and other eating utensils with a permanent marker, stickers, or duct tape, is an easy way to see which cutlery is yours.

Another way you can avoid cross-contamination is to eat gluten-free with your travel buddies when preparing food on vacation. This is easy to do if your companion(s) are also gluten-free. Instill the importance of your health and that you don't want anyone to have to take care of you or listen to you puking all night on their vacation. Let them know that ensuring your health and well-being while traveling benefits them as well as you!

ॐ 8 ॐ
SUPPLEMENTS YOU CAN TRAVEL WITH WHEN YOU'RE GLUTEN-FREE

Disclaimer: The following information is not intended to diagnose, prescribe, or dictate types of supplements you should take when you travel. These are supplements that I use for my personal care. Before using any supplement, check with your healthcare provider for any adverse side effects they could potentially cause to your health or could possibly interfere with other medications you may be currently taking.

A BIT OF PERSONAL HISTORY

For several years, starting in 1998, I owned a health food store in the town where I lived in Florida. I really enjoyed assisting my clients in choosing supplements and brands to help them achieve their health goals. My clients' health issues ranged from the common cold to ringworm to cancer and much other different chronic and acute health issues. I could almost always recommend a supplement for my client and assist them in feeling better.

Although I didn't have a degree in the medical field, I was

often asked if I was a doctor because of my extensive knowledge of supplements. I researched and read many articles and books and kept up on the latest supplements to make sure my clients were getting the best suggestions when they walked into my door. Although I could not prescribe or diagnose pharmaceutical medicines, knowing I enjoyed helping my clients to better health and was my "why" for going to work in the morning.

Even with this exposure to supplements and the wide variety of health issues of my clients, back in the late 1990s, I hardly ever heard of people who were Celiac. I had only a fundamental understanding of this issue. I carried gluten-free pasta for those who could not eat regular pasta. Celiac disease was not well researched, diagnosed, or tested for in individuals during this time. As you know, Celiac disease, gluten-intolerance, and gluten sensitivity are a well-recognized and prevalent issue in American society today. As a result, there are different supplements you can take to lessen the effects and fallout of eating gluten when you are Celiac.

Taking these supplements does not minimize the attack your immune system will take on your body. Do not read this information assuming that taking these supplements will make "cheating" better. When you have Celiac, having a "cheat" day, snack or meal will always wreak massive amounts of damage on your small intestine, digestive system, muscles, and joints. The damage caused by Celiac disease to your small intestine is cumulative. A little "snack" could take weeks or months for your body to repair. Understand that taking these supplements should NEVER be used as an excuse to eat gluten. The only way to avoid cancers and secondary issues resulting from Celiac disease is to eat a completely gluten-free diet without cheating.

We'll explore the different supplements that I use when I travel. I take these tried and true supplements on every travel adventure to use for Celiac, general stomach upset, intestinal upset, motion sickness, or your general digestive health.

CHARCOAL

Charcoal is traditionally used to clean up toxins in your system. Veterinarians often use charcoal when animal patients have digested a non-digestible or toxic item. The easiest way to use charcoal is by taking capsules. I use charcoal when I feel that I've been cross-contaminated or glutened when eating out.

I also take this supplement when, let's say, my digestive system wants to get rid of solid waste faster than usual. I've found that charcoal helps to bind solid food particles in the intestine to transit them through your system while stopping the dehydration risk from diarrhea at the same time. Drink lots of water when you take charcoal for the most benefit from this supplement. Additionally, stop taking charcoal when your bowel movements become your "normal" because you can run the risk of constipation if you continue to take charcoal with normal stools.

PROBIOTICS

You hear so much about probiotics in the natural health and supplement realm concerning digestion disorders and issues. Why? Recently, scientists have found out that we have neural (brain) tissue in our digestive tract. Yes, we have brains in our intestines. Although this sounds bizarre, I remember many clients at my health food store told me they felt better when taking probiotics and cleaned up their diet. Common words my clients would say to me were they felt, "Less fuzzy," "more clear," and "more focused." I've also heard of people having fewer symptoms from their Schizophrenia when they have cleaned up their diet and taken probiotics.

Having neural tissue in your digestive tract brings even more importance to taking care of this fragile system, which breaks down your food and gives you nutrients to survive. Most recently, scientists have found a link between your gut and your immune system. Not surprising to Celiac, the immune system can protect or wreak havoc on your own body if your immune system incorrectly attacks your body.

Probiotics are the good bacteria found in your digestive system. On average, we are made of five to seven pounds of bacteria, depending on how tall you are and your body volume. Your gut consists of many types of microbes that live within your body. Microbes are living creatures so small you can only see them with a microscope. The most prolific microbes are bacteria.

Similar to a superhero movie, there are two main types of bacteria: good bacteria and harmful bacteria. Healthy individuals have trillions of different species of good bacteria in their digestive system with tiny amounts of bad bacteria.

WHAT DO THE GOOD BACTERIA DO?

- Assist in digesting food
- Kill bad bacteria
- Do away with other invaders in your digestive tract
- Keep your immune system up and running well
- Absorb liquids in our large intestine when we eat food or drink

An individual with an overload of harmful bacteria can become very sick and die. My father, when in the hospital for adenocarcinoma, ended up with C. diff, an overgrowth of the harmful bacteria. Clostridium difficile causes explosive diarrhea, severe dehydration, increased white blood cell count, rapid heart rate, and fever, among other symptoms. I remember his heart rate (not blood pressure) would rise above 200 when he used the bathroom as this condition is also painful. So how did my dad get so sick? From the use of long-term antibiotics in the hospital.

But you don't have to be in a hospital to get C. diff. Anyone using antibiotics, especially Clindamycin, can get C. diff in as little as 5 days. This is why it's so important to take probiotics when taking antibiotics as antibiotics kill all the bacteria - good or bad - which leaves a lot of real estate in your gut for harmful bacteria, such as C. diff. and many other species of harmful bacteria, to take hold in your gut and make you sick.

Taking Probiotics

When taking probiotics, make sure to take them two hours after you take your antibiotic. Taking them with your antibiotic will render your antibiotic useless and kill all the good bacteria in your supplement. If you have a prescription probiotic, take your probiotic as instructed.

Probiotics come in many different forms: liquid, powder, chewable, tablet, and capsule. For travel, pre-packaged individual servings in capsules or chewable work best. My healthcare provider suggested 50 billion probiotics per serving, with several different strains of probiotics for daily use. There are many different brands of probiotics you can use to restore gut biome. I am currently using Renew Life probiotics and Garden of Eden, which you can find in many health foods stores.

When using probiotics, you want to use a supplement with different bacteria strains to give your system a variety of friendly helpers. Each species of good bacteria does a specific job in your gut. Taking these friendly bacteria protects you when using an antibiotic and keeps your digestive system in balance and assists your immune system in keeping harmful bacteria at a minimum in your gut.

Ginger

Good ole' ginger - a great digestive aide used for morning sickness, motion sickness, and any time your stomach isn't feeling well, especially when you've accidentally eaten gluten. With no harmful side effects to speak of, you can easily take this supplement with you in the form of ginger candy, lozenges, tea, capsules, or even fresh ginger root. Although the latter is the best, especially for making tea, fresh ginger may be a bit hard to transport while traveling. Additionally, fresh ginger can be tagged and taken away by TSA as a fresh fruit that can transport bugs or other unwanted lives across country borders.

My preferred form of ginger, which is free of sugar, is ginger lozenges when I travel. As the name implies, ginger lozenges are tablets of ginger that you can place in your mouth and let dissolve. These are the most accessible form of ginger to take with you as they don't melt, have a long shelf life, are easy to transport, and don't require water to swallow the supplement.

I usually take ginger lozenges in a small vitamin container that has only ginger lozenges in the container. This way, I can quickly grab a lozenge on a plane ride if I encounter turbulence, when I've accidentally ingested gluten, or I'm feeling nauseous on a car ride. Now Foods makes a great lozenge which I take with me every time I travel, even on long car trips!

Protein Shakes

I commonly carry protein bars and shakes with me,

whether I'm working on the go or traveling. These two types of supplements are an easy way to eat a clean and nutritious snack at any time of the day or night! There are several different protein bases to choose from: soy, whey, hemp, pea protein, milk (casein), or a combination of these proteins.

Since I've found pea protein to be the most easily digestible for my system, I use the type of protein to make my smoothie in the mornings. Additionally, I like that my morning breakfast smoothie is my most eco-friendly meal of the day. In addition to pea protein from Now Foods, I also add oats, a serving of frozen fruit, almond milk (or another plant-based milk), a scoop of Orgain Collagen Peptides, and a scoop of Gemini Foods Superboost Smoothie Mix. This combination works well for me; however, I've found it quite hard to mix these and bring them in a double Ziploc bag. Scooping out the protein is a challenge as static on the plastic bag attracts my protein's powders, creating a mess when reopened.

When I travel, I found that it's most convenient to use single-serving protein powder pouches. Be sure to check the carbohydrate count (for excessive carbohydrates due to added sugar) and read the sweetener ingredients to make sure the company does not add artificial sweeteners. I usually find a protein that is pea-based and has mixed greens and probiotics. Additionally, I travel with a shaker bottle, which can be easily carried in my travel backpack.

I've found eating protein drinks a lifesaver after getting off a red-eye flight. For travelers who haven't taken a red-eye flight, this is an overnight flight that usually leaves the airport between 11:00 pm and midnight and arrives at the destination between 5:30 am, and 7:30 am. I like these flights because you get to your destination with an entire day to have fun. Am I tired? Yup! But it's well worth the lack of sleep to have a whole day of travel when you land. Here's the bad news.

Many of the food vendors close from 11 pm until 6:00 am. You're out of luck to grab breakfast at the airport before 6am. No matter, I've only found one or two places I can actually eat a safe breakfast at an airport in all the travels I've taken. This is where your incredibly healthy, safe, and convenient protein drink comes in handy!

Make sure to store your single protein serving inside your shaker bottle. Take your protein packet out, find a water fountain that caters to water bottles. These are easy to spot as they have the blue water bottle on the splash back of the fountain. Fill your shaker bottle with about four or five ounces of water.

Add your protein drink. CAUTION: Do NOT, I repeat, DO NOT, put your protein first. If you do, the water will sit around the dry protein, sticking it to your shaker's bottom.

After adding water, add your protein and shake well - and I mean well! If you don't shake your protein drink vigorously, you will end up with a clumpy protein drink. While this may not harm you, I can tell you from experience that this is not the best texture to drink.

Good fortune comes your way if you have gotten off your red-eye flight and can find a store that carries single-serving plant-based milk! Be warned, you will pay a premium price of around $3 for a single serving. However, this does create a better taste and texture for your morning smoothie and adds more protein and nutrients.

Protein Bars

Traveling with protein bars can be tricky because you have to clearly read the ingredients and see what type of coating the bar contains. If the bar has a coating that is chocolate or quickly melts, do not choose that bar to bring along on trips or to pack in your bag. I've had

THE GUIDE TO TRAVELING GLUTEN FREE

protein bars melt. When opened, splash that delicious coating all over you and anyone standing within 6 feet of your location. Melted bars can also wreak havoc on clothing and other items packed inside your carry-on or suitcase.

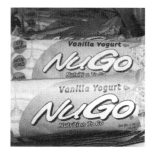

Protein bars come in many different shapes, sizes, and flavors. Back in the day, in the early 90s, protein bars were few and far between and were carbohydrate-based as the dietary fad back then was to ramp up on carbs before and after your workout. Wow, our healthy dietary eating habits have changed 180 since then!

Always read the ingredients of your protein bar as they range significantly from company to company, brand to brand. Even within brands, you can find different protein bases. Protein bases used for bars include meat, egg, whey, milk (casein), soy, rice, pea protein, and hemp. I've found it best for my digestive system to stay away from the egg and dairy-based bars.

I highly recommend trying different flavors and bars before you travel to find a protein bar you like. Also, check for certified gluten-free bars, as some companies have certified their bars to be safe for Celiac! Many bars, however, have allergen warnings. If you or the person you are buying bars for has an allergy, make sure to read the allergy warnings before purchasing it.

PROTEIN COOKIES

One of my favorite new gluten-free food discoveries is that protein cookies taste like a real cookie, with one big exception - they are actually good for you! My favorite is

NuGo protein cookies with peanut butter. I also love their chocolate chip version. Besides tasting great, NuGo brand is also vegetarian and certified gluten-free - it's a win-win for travel food.

Additionally, protein cookies usually do not have a coating that melts, making them excellent travel food. They are slender and fit easily into your backpack or carry-on purse or bag. Remember that red-eye I talked about previously? Yup, that little kid inside of me loves that I can still eat a cookie for breakfast. Luckily, protein cookies are much healthier than the Chips Ahoy! cookies I would eat growing up on Saturday mornings while watching cartoons.

Check out different brands as there are many types of protein cookies on the market. Be aware, read the ingredients and the nutrition label to see if they have added sugar. I don't buy from companies or products that have added sugar because that isn't a healthy, high-quality product. Again, try different brands BEFORE you travel, so you can choose a cookie that works for you! You don't want to bring a cookie on your trip to find out that you dislike the taste.

Enzymes

Enzymes are what breaks down our food so we can absorb vitamins and minerals from what we eat. These are essential for overall health, especially gut health. Your body can produce some enzymes, and others you get from food. Lacking in the production of or being deficient in certain enzymes can wreak havoc on your body. Enzymes are essential for proper digestion and absorption of macronutrients. Each enzyme will break down a specific macromolecule:

- Papain, Bromelain and Protease breaks down protein

- Amylase for starch
- Cellulase breaks down vegetable fiber
- Invertase dissects sucrose into fructose and glucose
- Lipase disintegrates fat
- Lactase dissects milk sugar
- Glucoamylase breaks down sugars that are attached to starches

I use enzymes to assist my body in breaking down food since I have pancreatic insufficiency. Your pancreas secretes many of the proteins you use to break down your food since my pancreas isn't very efficient.

If you eat gluten, your body has to go through the process of digesting it, then it wreaks havoc on your body. To expedite this process, I use Doctor's Best Gluten Rescue. This formula has a plant protein enzyme blend to break down gluten more quickly so it can move through your system faster.

The last time I was accidentally glutened, a waitress gave me a wheat crust pizza even though I told her I was Celiac and allergic to gluten. Also, I told her I couldn't eat gluten because of medical reasons. She somehow wholly forgot this but remembered me saying I wanted Olive Oil on my crust instead of tomatoes. Three bites in, I wondered if it was really gluten-free, and when I asked the waitress - the look on her face told me it wasn't.

Usually, I would ask before I eat; however, I was traveling in my car all day and was super hungry. My hungry stomach took over my brain, and I accidentally ate wheat.

Luckily, I had my Gluten Rescue and other travel supplements in the car. I took Gluten Rescue, along with probiotics, charcoal, and my Naltrexone (listen to Episode #82 for information about this compounded medication). Amazingly enough, I didn't puke my guts up for the next six hours. However, I did suffer from horrid joint and muscle pain the next day while canyoneering for six hours, but out of the two evils, I'll take that one any day!

Arnica

This little flower is created and used in homeopathic medicine for hundreds of years. The best pain reliever for sore muscles and joints and is a lifesaver for me as a writer for my full-time regular job. Having painful hand joints is not a great combination when you're typing 5,000 words a day.

You can take Arnica tablets in different doses, use Arnica in cream or oil, and apply them topically. Arnica is added to some joint supplements in capsule form as well. I most often use Arnica in massage oil from Weleda, which smells fantastic and feels great. The other Arnica topical supplement I would recommend is Topricin cream. A bit pricey. However, this cream is well worth its price in gold. I've been able to skip using over the counter anti-inflammatories when using this on my achy hand joints or sore muscles.

I prefer to use creams and oils instead of over-the-counter pain medication as I have an allergy to ibuprofen. Additionally, I'll take the option to put medicine on my skin instead of through my digestive tract. This is one less irritating factor for my digestive organs.

SUPPLEMENTS FOR SLEEP

I didn't know that not being able to get through the night with sufficient sleep was a symptom of the auto-immune disease until I read this on a medical website. I have been having issues with sleeping for several years, even before my experience with auto-immune disease. Going to sleep is a piece of cake, staying asleep through the night and not waking up at 3 am until 4 am or so is the part that I grapple with on a nightly basis.

There are several different supplements you can use for sleep. Make sure to check with your healthcare provider as some of these supplements can have interactions with specific prescriptions. I would not recommend taking these during the day as they all make you sleepy.

I use different supplements to stay asleep at night and rotate them out, so my body doesn't become immune to the effects. Valerian, kava kava, California Poppy and CBD are supplements that I use for inflammation, sleep, and sore muscles.

These herbs and other supplements listed below can be found and used on their own; or in combination with each other. Personally, I like combination formulas for sleep, as I feel they work better for my body.

Valerian Root

This root works way better than it smells. Valerian root smells like you took last night's dinner, threw it in a swamp, took the water surrounding this mess the next day, and bottled this concoction.

With large amounts of calcium and magnesium, it's no wonder this herb is helpful for sleep. I've also used Valerian Root for muscle cramps, backache, and other issues associated with sore muscles. You can find this in tincture (with or without alcohol), capsules, or pill form. If you can't stomach the smell, I would go with capsules first. I would also recommend getting a standardized Valerian Root supplement as you know exactly how much you are getting with each serving.

. . .

Melatonin

Melatonin is a hormone our body creates to sleep through the night. Melatonin, along with many other hormones and chemicals, isn't produced as efficiently as we age. We are then left with an insufficient quantity of hormones. As a result, we can be left with a low level of Melatonin - with the possible side effect of not sleeping throughout the night.

I've tried Melatonin, and unfortunately, for me, this supplement gives me a hangover in the morning. According to the nurse-physician I used several years ago, this happens to 20% of the population. Of course, my body usually has the most non-statistical reaction to most everything, including Melatonin.

However, many of my friends have used Melatonin with excellent results. One of my friends was able to sleep longer and better sleep quality when using this supplement. Many people start with a low 3mg dose to see how this amount affects your sleep. If you take Melatonin and feel like you have a hangover, stop using this supplement. However, if you feel good the next day, you may have found a supplement to help you sleep through the night!

Passionflower

Passionflower is an herb that is used for calming anxiety and sleep. I have only found this supplement mostly intermixed with other herbs in a combination formula.

Kava Kava

A fantastic root used for muscle relaxation, I've used Kava as a tea before bed to help with achy and sore muscles. I have also used Kava for PMS symptoms as well as a sleep aid. I really like combining Kava Kava with Valerian root for deep sleep and relaxation.

California Poppy

It is a relatively new supplement to hit the natural food scene. I really like this supplement for its ability to keep me sleeping through the night and its anti-anxiety effect on my well-being.

CBD

CBD is the latest craze on the health food scene today, and with good reason. CBD is the cannabinoid from the hemp plant. It is not marijuana, nor does it have the same side effects as marijuana. You can receive the pain-relieving benefit of CBD without having the side effects of the narcotic drug. I really love CBD muscle balms, as they are wonderful for relieving sore muscles.

DIFFERENT FORMS OF SUPPLEMENTS

Whether you use a capsule, liquid, dissolvable tablet, or a tablet, you have to swallow, use what works best for you. For me, I've found that liquid tinctures work best; however, liquids aren't always the best choice for the sake of time and convenience.

Please take special care to make sure you are using a tincture, especially with children or pregnant, to read the ingredients on the bottle first. Some are made using alcohol to extract the herbal properties, and while OK for adults, you do not want to use a liquid herbal that contains alcohol for children. There are many different children's lines, including Herbs for Kids that are all alcohol-free and safe for children.

Both are just as effective, please be sure to use only alcohol-free tinctures for children.

TAKING AND ORGANIZING MULTIPLE SUPPLEMENTS

If you take three or more supplements at a time, definitely try out a vitamin case. These are sold at supermarkets, online and in pharmacies. You can find them anywhere that prescriptions or supplements are sold.

I have one for morning and another for nighttime. My morning vitamin case has the daily vitamins I take for thyroid function, circulation, and digestive health. The nighttime vitamin case has my magnesium, valerian, kava, and other supplements I take at night for sleep. I refill these once a week and label the compartments for each day of the week. When I'm half asleep in the morning or tired at night, I can tell if I've taken my vitamins for the day and not make the mistake of taking them twice.

Although some vitamins and minerals can be toxic when overused, most people do not take vitamins in that high a quantity that they would see an adverse side effect. However, better to be safe than sorry, and I'm not a fan of waste. Invest in vitamin cases and take the hassle out of opening multiple bottles more than once a week! Additionally, these are also super convenient when traveling. They take up a small amount of space in your luggage - much less than several bottles. When packing for travel, make sure to wrap your vitamin case in a Ziploc - they can easily open up and spill in transit.

9

SO YOU'VE BEEN GLUTENED, NOW WHAT?

Depending on your reaction to gluten, there are several supplements you can take and methods you can use to lessen the effect of gluten on your system. Listen in to Episode #64 Travel Supplements for Celiacs, where I share the supplements I take with me on my travel adventures. These methods may not work for everyone and remember to always check with a healthcare provider to make sure these supplements are safe for you to take.

STEP #1: DETERMINE WHAT TYPE OF GLUTEN YOU'VE BEEN POISONED WITH.

I've found that fried gluten is the worst for me and means I'll most likely be puking for hours. I can set my watch for 15 minutes, and I know if I feel sick, that means I need to get back to my house ASAP, or I'll be puking in the car.

Suppose I've eaten a piece of bread, depending on the type of bread and the flour source. In that case, I can usually take several supplements and not get horribly ill. However, I will be in pain for the next two to three days, especially when walking upstairs. My quadriceps muscles are hugely affected by pain and stiffness when I've consumed gluten.

If someone wasn't careful, and cross-contamination happens, I usually don't know until the next day. At this point, I have bad joint and muscle pain, and my stomach will feel sick, but I won't be vomiting.

STEP #2: DRINK LOTS AND LOTS OF WATER

At this point, you have gluten in your system. If I know that the gluten is still in my stomach, I'll purposely vomit so that the protein doesn't go through my entire digestive tract. While extremely uncomfortable in the short term, I feel that this does less damage overall than if I let the gluten protein go into my gut. When gluten gets loose in my body, I have a more extreme reaction where I'm sick for several days.

No matter what, flushing your body with water is always a good idea when toxins have been added to your system. Water will help move the gluten through your body faster and help yourself get any by-products of the toxins out of your body through urination.

You can also sit in a heated sauna or steam room as sweating out the toxins is also a known way to get the poison out of your system. Sitting outside in the sun, soaking in a tub of hot water with Epsom salts or sitting outside on a warm sunny day in a lounge chair, has helped my stiffness immensely when my joints flare-up. Make sure to do what makes YOU feel comfortable. If you feel "pukey" the heat may make you feel worse. Remember to listen to your body!

STEP #3: TAKE NALTREXONE

In Episode #82, I chat with Amie and Rory of Peak Medical about Naltrexone. Ever since I've taken this compounded prescription medicine, my pain level in my joints has significantly reduced! Before taking this drug, I would have many mornings in a row where it would take me almost a half hour to get out of bed as a result of pain and stiffness. I've taken Naltrexone every day for more than six months now, and I know when I've forgotten to take it! Now, however, I'm almost entirely pain-free, except for when I eat corn. This drug is a significant game-changer for me, and it's one of the first things I take if I've been glutened. Talk to your doctor about taking Naltrexone; if they aren't receptive to it, I'd recommend calling Amie and Rory at Peak Medical 435-602-1034 for a complimentary consultation.

STEP #4: CHARCOAL

Charcoal is a supplement that I take any time I've been poisoned with gluten. Charcoal has been used for hundreds of years in human history. Veterinarians use charcoal when an animal has eaten something that makes them sick. Charcoal binds to the toxins in your body and carries them out safely. I always keep charcoal in abundance in my home and start taking it immediately when I get diarrhea!

STEP #5: PROBIOTICS

You may be thinking, wow, there are so many things to take when you get glutened, and believe me, that is the case! However, I'd rather take a bunch of supplements and limit the amount of pain and anguish.

Probiotics have been a popular supplement for decades

and have recently seen a resurgence in popularity. They are the good bacteria in your gut. Without them, we would not be able to live. When we accidentally eat gluten, this throws off the balance of good bacteria in our body and wipes out many of the good guys we have that support our digestion, immune system, and brain. Taking probiotics if you've eaten gluten is an excellent way to replace any of your lost defenders.

STEP #6: EAT FERMENTED FOODS

Definitely, don't eat if you're horribly puking! When you're feeling better, eating foods that are fermented also increases the viability of your gut's good bacteria, restoring your health faster. Examples include pickled foods, Kombucha, and any food fermented with vinegar. Ensure the food is gluten-free, as there are fermented foods containing soy sauce, which has gluten.

STEP #7: REST

Many of us try to push through when we're sick, which equates to taking the body an even longer time to recoup. Walking or stretching may be fine to do, but don't overwork yourself when you're sick. I find that walking is a great digestive aid and helps me to recover more quickly from a variety of different side effects from Celiac disease.

Heating pads are another world's greatest invention and work wonders for stomach cramps, back pain, and upset stomach. Heating pads are great for muscle cramping and calming your stomach after you've puked. Additionally, when you are resting, be sure to take off the heating pad if you're using one – you can quickly get burned sleeping with a heating pad.

Remember to always check with your healthcare physician or a licensed medical practitioner before starting a supplement. I've found them helpful in many different healing modalities. I believe they are a great asset to those of us with an auto-immune disease.

10

GLUTEN FREE TRAVEL COSMETICS

First, you find out that you can't eat 99% of the foods you love. THEN you find out that gluten could be in your toothpaste, shampoo, hair products, and body care! Really? Does gluten need to be in everything that you use throughout your day?

I was thrilled to find a safe and natural product line that does not contain gluten when I found Lemongrass Spa. Additionally, I found out that their entire product line is natural and free from over 100 chemicals; also, the business is female-owned, and they don't test on animals! Check out Episode #83, where I talk about my favorite Lemongrass Spa cosmetics. I'd highly recommend you listen to that episode if you haven't yet.

Added bonus - many of their amazing products also come in travel sizes and travel cases! Find fantastic hair products, skin conditioners, and their all-natural bug repellent in convenient 2 oz sizes. These fun-sized products are great to keep in your car, baby bag, or backpack and packing in your carry-on luggage for a plane ride!

Although this is not a list of the complete line of Lemongrass Spa products, the body care mentioned in this chapter are some of my favorite's I've used from this line.

I bought a few items and ended up becoming a consultant for Lemongrass Spa. Full disclosure: ordering from Lemongrass Spa links on my website at http://www.travelglutenfreepodcast.com, click on Travel Cosmetics. Purchases made on my associate page financially support my podcast. You get safe, amazing gluten-free cosmetics and, in return, get to support the information you love!

SPA PRODUCTS THAT ARE ECO FRIENDLY

Did you know the average amount of chemicals in your skincare? There are, on average, 25 chemicals in each of the cosmetics you use daily! That's right, you are putting an average of 25 chemicals onto the largest organ in your body - your skin. Two offenders with the highest toxins are lipstick at 33 toxins and sunscreen and body lotion at 32 toxins. These are two products I use every day, sometimes more than once a day! I'm thrilled that I've switched over to safer products.

Why is eco-friendly, non-toxic skincare vital to me? I have cancer in my family on both sides, low thyroid, and Celiac disease. I'm swapping out my skin and body care essentials I own now for lemongrass spa products.

CHEMICAL FREE HYDRATION FOR YOUR SKIN

Keeping skin hydrated, especially in dry climates, equates to using alcohol-free cosmetics and drinking lots of water. Make sure to read the labels of your current products. Do you see alcohol listed as one of the first three ingredients? That means that one of the three most substantial amounts of ingredients in your product is alcohol! Extremely drying to your skin, any product that claims hydration should definitely

NOT have alcohol as an ingredient. How can you hydrate if you're always drying out your skin by putting alcohol on it?

Hand sanitizer has loads of alcohol, which is why it dries out your hands. The purpose of hand sanitizer, however, is not to moisturize, but to kill germs. Besides alcohol, sanitizer can have many unhealthy chemicals, so I use Lemongrass Spa hand sanitizer. Take away the germs without adding noxious chemicals to your hands!

Besides my hands, I find my face is super hard to keep hydrated, especially overnight. Lemongrass Spa's Coconut Overnight Rehab Cream is a high moisture cream, applied at night, to rehydrate dry skin.

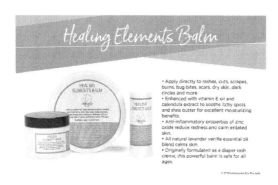

Healing Elements is a fantastic cream that keeps my super dry skin hydrated overnight as well. Besides being super-healing, it smells deliciously amazing! It's a heavy cream, with a texture like a salve. There's no doubt you have a protective layer between your skin and the elements when you put this on your skin. I've recently used this cream on a 23-inch surgical scar, and my surgeon was super impressed with how healed my scar was two weeks post-op. I've also used this on my hands, legs, arms, face, and lips in the winter. There are very few places on my body where I haven't used this amazing cream!

You can get this in travel size or a stick that is super easy to use and is not considered a liquid! My dog Lily loves to taste when I'm applying this to my skin after a shower. Many cancer patients have used this cream to heal their sensitive, burned, and dry skin from chemotherapy or radiation.

If you are currently undergoing cancer treatment, please contact me through my website http://www.travelglutenfreepodcast.com on my contact page. Lemongrass Spa offers complementary cancer care packages to those going through cancer treatment. I'd be happy to have them ship you a complimentary skincare package!

Ultra Hydrating Body Cream is a concentrated cream that is a bit lighter than Healing Elements. Ultra Hydrating Cream is great for everyday use on any type of dry skin. It's unscented, gluten, and chemical-free. I have very sensitive skin, and this cream has never bothered my skin in any way. I would recommend this cream for kids who have sensory issues and people who don't like strong smells as it does not have a funny unscented fragrance or any type of abrasives. It's very smooth and lightweight. This comes in a travel size as well!

Your nails take a beating when you're living your outdoor experience. Lemongrass Spa's ultra-hydrating nail balm will give your nails a layer of protection while keeping your nails and skin hydrated. No need to worry about having dry, cracked, or damaged nails at the end of your camping trip! Grab the travel-ready 2oz size or get the travel set with a stick and 2oz cream to keep in your backpack and travel bag!

TINTED SUNSCREEN - FORGO THE WHITE GLOW!

An essential element to any outdoor activity, many sunscreens have artificial perfumes or chemicals you don't want in your open pores, especially when you're outdoors swimming in a lake or natural body of water. Marine life definitely doesn't appreciate our chemicals in their environment either!

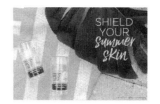

Lemongrass Spa tinted sunscreen is my absolute favorite sunscreen and the only one I wear on my face. The tint in the sunscreen prevents that cloudy white look from regular sunscreen. I've found this sunscreen prevents sunburn better than other, more expensive sunscreens I've put on my face. It's a no brainer when it comes to sunscreen for your face. In a stick, and not considered a liquid, Sunscreen Sport Stick is easy to transport and use wherever your next outdoor adventure takes you!

BUG-A-BOO INSECT REPELLENT

Also, in a 1 oz stick and not a liquid, the Bug-a-Boo insect repellent is easy to take along when traveling! Keep the bugs away with a natural alternative, formulated with skin-softening almond oil, beeswax, geranium essential oil, catnip essential oil, citronella, and cedarwood. It does not contain any DEET or chemically derived insecticides. Kid-safe and environmentally friendly.

If you're looking for a spray, grab Bug-a-Boo duo, sold in a convenient two-pack with a 4oz size for at home and a 2oz size for travel! Drop-in your backpack and carry along to reapply when hiking, at the beach, or enjoying a picnic at the park or in the backcountry.

Want both the stick and the liquid spray? The Bug-a-Bool Family Pack contains the duo spray with the 1oz stick for a bundled discounted price!

HAND CLEANLINESS WHILE TRAVELING

I carry my Lemon sorbet foaming liquid soap around in my purse with a small fun-sized foaming soap bottle from Lemongrass Spa, so I don't have to use toxic bathroom soap. Hand Sanitizer is essential for your everyday cleanliness when you are traveling!

GLUTEN-FREE COSMETICS TRAVEL SIZE SETS

Travel Skincare Set: Beautifully Balanced

Includes trial size Tea Tree Bar Soap, Tea Tree Cleansing Gel, Tea Tree Face Crème, Repair Water Gel, Charcoal Detox Facial Mask, packaged in a zipper logo bag with instruction card.

Travel Face Care Set: Anti-Aging

This travel sized anti-aging face kit contains a set of five trial-sized products in a clear cosmetic bag. Features Botanical Cleansing Gel, Vitamin C Serum, Botanical Face Crème, Hydrating Facial Polish and Hydrating Eye Crème.

Clean Slate Gift Set w/Travel Bag for Men

A gentleman deserves soft and healthy skin at home or on the go with the Clean Slate Gift Set. The Gift Set includes a Lotion Duo, a Bar Soap, an After Shave Splash, and a Deodorant in a gray zipper bag. Our Clean Slate Collection will keep him handsome and fresh from head to toe. Cedarwood and bay rum is mellowed with amber and citrus, reminiscent of the local barbershop's clean shave. 8 oz + 2 oz lotion duo, bar soap, 4 oz aftershave splash, 2 oz deodorant stick.

Cherry Almond Shampoo & Conditioner Pair 2 oz travel size

Stimulate your senses, while cleansing, softening and conditioning your hair with this 2 oz Cherry Almond

Shampoo and Conditioner pair. Great for all hair types, this invigorating duo is handcrafted with natural aloe vera, coconut oil, and d-panthenol to soothe the scalp, leaving hair refreshingly clean and touchable smooth. One 2 oz bottle of Shampoo and one 2 oz bottle of conditioner are packaged together in this set.

Travel Skincare Set: Naturally Radiant

This travel-friendly set contains a set of five trial-sized products in a clear cosmetic bag. Features Botanical Cleansing Gel, Hydrating Eye Creme, Hydrating Facial Polish, Coconut Rehab Creme, and Hydrating Facial Mask.

Travel Skincare Set: Charcoal Detox

Cleanse, exfoliate and detoxify your skin, for a refreshing facial experience. Kit includes travel-friendly Charcoal Detox Facial Soap, Charcoal Detox Facial Mask, Charcoal Detox Facial Polish, Tea Tree Face Crème, and Repair Eye Crème.

No matter which product you choose, you'll be so happy with your Lemongrass Spa purchase! To find out more about Lemongrass Spa products, visit my YouTube Channel, Travel Gluten Free Podcast Episode #83 or purchase Lemongrass Spa products directly from my site today! You can also sign up for Lemongrass Spa Newsletter featuring this month's sale items.

Lemongrass Spa offers

100% gluten-free

skin care,
body care and
makeup products.

11

HOW TO PACK YOUR GLUTEN FREE TRAVEL BAGS

Have you ever packed food in your suitcase and found it scattered all over your clothes and staining your luggage? Are you new to Celiac Disease and didn't know you had to pack food to safely eat when you travel? Many times, packing food, and the right type of food, makes traveling more carefree and easier. However, you need to pack the right kind of food and avoid packing certain items that will melt or explode!

Packing your bags, whether you are going on a cruise, road trip, or airplane ride, requires a bit more planning when you are traveling gluten-free. Each one of these types of travel will have you packing a bit more or less in the different kinds of bags, you are bringing on your adventure.

With proper organization and the right travel tools and accessories, you can enjoy your gluten-free vacation without worry or anxiety!

PACKING YOUR BAGS FOR A CRUISE

From a food standpoint, cruises are the easiest way to travel when you are on a restricted or specialty diet. You will be eating so much food, you don't have to worry about carrying a lot of food. You can return to your ship to eat lunch or dinner, then continue your vacation adventure!

Pack two or three snacks and your own reusable water bottle when you are out and visit your port of call. Additionally, make sure to pack what you need if you travel by plane or car to your port of call. See Chapter 12 to find out what to pack in your bags when you are traveling by air.

ROAD TRIP FOOD

When you're on a road trip, you have access to more gluten-free foods. Likewise, you can create your own schedule and stop when you are hungry, go food shopping, or find a new adventure you've never had the opportunity to do before. You won't have to pack food in your suitcase or clothing bag for a road trip as you can take along a cooler and reusable shopping bags, which you can pack with enough food for your trip.

I suggest packing two to three snacks per day per gluten-free person. Additionally, I like to pack coconut water and other drinks that are flavored in a cooler. Buying drinks at gas stations can quickly add up to a significant expense, and this helps to keep costs down.

If you stop for sightseeing, make sure to bring a shoulder bag with snacks for each gluten-free person. You can also pack shelf-stable drinks in cardboard containers. While they may not be cold, you can be sure they are safe. You don't want to put cold containers in your bag as they will sweat and get the contents of your bag wet.

TRAVEL BAGS FOR AIR TRAVEL

See Chapter 12 for details on TSA restrictions and what you can and can't bring on an airplane. Packing for air travel depends highly on what airports you will be flying in and out of, how long you are traveling and how many stops you have to your destination.

The most crucial detail to always remember is that you can't bring outside liquids over 3oz per bottle into an airport, with few exceptions, such as baby formula and medication. Security will make you throw it out, and you will have lost that item. Make sure to check the TSA website, located in chapter 12 for up to date information on the latest TSA rules.

PACK SINGLE SERVE OR PREPACKAGED FOOD

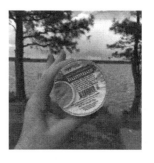

I really dislike buying single-serve food because of the expense and the extra packaging, except for travel.

Single serving sizes create a much more relaxed travel experience for you, especially for children, as you can quickly dispose of leftovers without repacking food. Repacking food, especially when traveling by air, can end up leaving a big mess or crumbling into pieces to the point where it's not edible. Remember, gluten-free food tends to be dry because it lacks gluten, and gluten gives food elasticity. Exposing gluten-free food to air will turn your food from yummy to concrete quickly.

Buy food that's prepackaged, especially when you are traveling by air. Using sandwich or quart-sized bags, pack snacks for each day or pack a few of the same snacks in each bag.

Now you can easily find your food and eat what you'd like to have when traveling without worrying about finding safe food.

Definitely avoid food with oils or liquids, if possible, as they can leak. Oils can stain, ruin and wreak havoc on bottle labels, clothing, and the lining of your luggage.

When I pack in my suitcase, I don't pack my liquid protein drinks, even in my carry on as they are larger than the allowed liquid limit. However, I do pack protein powder in single servings. I've tried double bagging the powder in plastic bags, yet; the static from the protein gets stuck to the bags and creates a mess. You will end up throwing out more packaging with single-serve, but when you're traveling, this is a side effect of eating safely. I'm an avid recycler at home. When I travel as much as possible, it balances out the single-serving trash created when I visit.

You can also pack single-serve protein powder, protein cookies, or bars in a bag in your suitcase. These foods are an easy way to get healthy and safe protein if I can't eat what is available. Make sure to read the labels carefully to avoid any other foods you may not be able to eat. Check out Chapter 14, where I list some of my favorite gluten-free travel snacks and foods, many of which are corn, soy, and dairy-free.

USING ZIPLOC BAGS FOR CARRYING FOOD

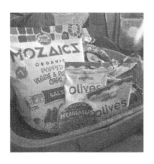

I'm a colossal recycler, and I don't like using a lot of plastic. However, using two plastic bags when packing food in your suitcase is definitely a reasonable precaution. If one of your snacks explodes in your luggage, two plastic bags are way better in containing the mess than one. TSA agents can also look through your bag, touching the outside bag, leaving the inside bag untouched!

In addition to using Ziploc bags, I also use packing cubes in my luggage. I use cubes for underwear and food every time I travel. Why? After the fourth time, I realized that I had a love letter from the TSA agents that they were touching all my clothing and looking through my bag. Packing cubes are a great way to keep your clothing "untouched" by agents checking your bag.

If you have a question on how to pack your bag, feel free to contact me via my contact form on my website or through Instagram @travelglutenfreepodcast, and I'll be glad to help you with your travel packing!

12
TRAVEL BY AIR

Looking to travel by air, but not sure what to do or how to pack for your next adventure on a plane? Check out these tips to make your next airline trip more gluten-free friendly!

AIRPORT FOOD: TAKING A BIG CHANCE

Many eating establishments in airports do not have adequately trained staff concerning food prep for those with allergies or medical conditions. Pre-packaged food, especially with a certified gluten-free label, is your best choice to buy from a small food stand or bookstore in an airport.

Fast food restaurants aren't generally safe to eat, except for Jersey Mike's and the waffle fries at Chick-Fil-A.

Sit down restaurants have a better protocol when it comes to serving gluten-free food. Usually, I like going to smaller, family-owned businesses; however, when I'm at an airport, I like to frequent chain restaurants with allergy protocols. This gives me peace-of-mind that I MOST -likely won't be sick on the airplane ride ahead of me.

Whatever airport you are at, if you are going to eat there, go to the information booth and ask them to list restaurants that serve gluten-free foods. Atlanta, Salt Lake City, and a few other airports I've been to have listings that show which restaurants are safe to eat.

Additionally, you can also use the Find Me Gluten Free app inside an airport. It has restaurants listed in the app. Usually, it will contain the terminal the restaurant is located in. If you're unsure, you can call the eating establishment from the airport and ask about their location.

OMG: GOING THROUGH AIRPORT SECURITY WITH FOOD!

I've been gluten-free for several years. At first, it was easy to get food through airline security as long as I had it in a clear bag inside my backpack.

I'm not quite sure what happened, but I've been tagged to have my bag searched with my food more than half of the time I go through security in the past couple of years. I've also had my checked luggage searched several times when I've packed food on my checked bag. Airport security will leave you a lovely little note on black paper telling you they searched your bag. What a lovely calling card!

I've had agents who were pretty cool when they had to check my carry-on bag. Usually, I wear my Travel Gluten-Free t-shirt when I'm traveling, and I tell people I'm gluten-free. Duh, if you haven't read my t-shirt? And I continue to educate them on Celiac disease, including the depth of sickness, which incurs upon ingesting gluten. One agent said, "No, wonder you carry your own food, can you even eat-out?"

HOW TO PACK YOUR GLUTEN FREE TRAVEL BAGS WHEN FLYING

Airplane packing can be really challenging, especially if you're traveling with children. Of course, as we know, you definitely want to make sure you pack enough snacks for each person per day of your vacation, plus snacks for the airplane. If you are traveling a red-eye flight, remember you have minimal breakfast options. Many of those options are not safe for Celiac at the airport.

When traveling by red-eye, I will pack two snacks, a protein cookie from NuGo, a protein shaker bottle, and a single pack of protein. Put your single package of protein inside the shaker bottle. You may have to fold the protein in half to fit. Next, put the shaker bottle in your backpack or carry-on.

Always use a backpack or a carry-on bag with a zipper or other enclosure that is easy to access and will keep your food from spilling on the airplane floor or in the overhead bin. Make sure your bag will fit underneath your seat.

I travel with an Osprey Commuter backpack that is designed for travel and safety. I would highly recommend spending the extra money on a high-quality backpack that will fit your snacks, water or shaker bottle, and your travel purse.

WHY I LOVE MY TRAVEL PURSE

My travel purse looks like a mini backpack with three main compartments. It's about 8" high and 3" wide, and I can stuff lip balm, hand sanitizer, a small wallet, my ID, and other essentials in my travel purse. Additionally, I can fit my travel purse inside my backpack. Now I officially have one carry-on that I can take out and use on the plane without having to put my essentials in a large carry-on bag.

DOMESTIC TRAVEL WITH LIQUIDS

The carefree days of travel where you could walk through an airport with a baby bag full of creams, water bottles, and regular-sized bottles of cosmetics are long gone. Today, you have to be a savvy traveler when you plan to travel by air, especially if you aren't going to check your luggage. TSA has strict rules about the total amount of liquids you can bring onto a plane in your checked baggage and the amount of liquid for each item.

Remember, this is for carry-on only! If you are planning to check luggage, I would highly recommend putting your cosmetic bag in your checked baggage. This way, you can avoid the hassle of TSA rummaging through your bags and taking out your liquid to a separate bin.

Remember the 3-1-1 travel rule for liquids: one quart-sized bag of liquids, aerosols, gels, creams, and pastes through the checkpoint. Each item is limited to 3.4 ounces (100 milliliters).

The TSA website states, "You are allowed to bring a quart-sized bag of liquids, aerosols, gels, creams, and pastes in your carry-on bag and through the checkpoint. These are limited to travel-sized containers that are 3.4 ounces (100 milliliters) or less per item. Placing these items in the small bag and separating from your carry-on baggage facilitates the screening process. Pack items that are in containers larger than 3.4 ounces or 100 milliliters in checked baggage.

Any liquid, aerosol, gel, cream, or paste that alarms during screening will require additional screening."

Except for baby food and medications, all other liquids must be 3.4oz or smaller and fit in a quart-sized bag. Remember, use Ziploc brand bags as these are sturdier than generic bags. Sure, you'll pay $2 more for Ziploc, but isn't that an excellent investment for protecting your entire suitcase of clothing from getting soaked with shampoo, soap, or toothpaste?

WHEN DO I HAVE TO TAKE OUT MY LIQUIDS OR COMPUTER FROM MY CARRY-ON BAG?

TSA changes these rules quite frequently. I've been on two different flights in the same month. One time I went to the airport they required liquids and computers out of my carry-on and into a separate bin and the other time I left them in my bag without a problem.

I believe it depends on how slow, fast, or backed up the TSA agents are when or if you need to take items out of your bag. Getting a travel or commuter backpack is key to rolling through the TSA checkpoint smoothly. These bags have a separate zipper compartment where you can take out your computer without having to open your bag's central space. Find out the most up-to-date TSA information about liquids on their website https://bit.ly/3g36bzf

INTERNATIONAL TRAVEL WITH LIQUIDS

TSA rule and regulations state: "You may carry duty free liquids in secure, tamper-evident bags, more than 3.4 oz or 100 ml in your carry-on bag if:

- The duty-free liquids were purchased internationally, and you are traveling to the United States with a connecting flight.
- The liquids are packed in a transparent, secure, tamper-evident bag by the retailer and do not show

signs of tampering when presented to TSA for screening.
- The original receipt for the liquids is present and the purchase was made within 48 hours."

"The items inside the secure, tamper-evident bags must be screened and cleared. Any item that alarms or is unable to be screened will not be permitted in your carry-on bag. We recommend packing all liquids, gels, and aerosols that are over 3.4 oz or 100 ml in your checked baggage, even if they are in a secure, tamper-evident bag."

INBOUND INTERNATIONAL FLIGHTS

Traveling internationally is definitely more energy-intensive than going domestic. You have to wait in more and longer lines. If there's an issue with your passport, then you are redirected to a small office where they look at your passport and ask you a bunch of questions before they let you get onto your flight.

How do I know this? When I had back to back trips returning from Austria and departing to Orlando. I accidentally left my passport on the flight coming home from Austria. I then had to purchase a new passport. Apparently, when you do that, you're put on a "list" of non-trustworthy people as I've had issues getting through international travel.

PACK AND PLAN AHEAD

Pack your checked bag with snacks for your trip that will stand up to heat and airline handling. We know how the airlines are going to throw around our bags, open them up and rummage around inside our suitcase! Pack your snacks, even if they are single-serving, inside two Ziplock bags, then pack all your snacks into one large Ziploc for extra protection.

If your bag gets marked for a search, TSA agents will rummage through your luggage, making a mess of your food. Keeping them in a see-through Ziplock keeps them organized and safe while letting the TSA security agent see what is in your bag. You can also put a message inside your bag (facing out) that you are Celiac and have a food allergy. People don't understand Celiac, so we make it easy for them by saying we have an "allergy." The TSA agent can read your note and is more likely to leave your food alone.

Make sure not to pack liquids over 3.4 oz inside your carry-on suitcase as the agent will make you throw them out. This has happened to me in London. It wasn't a fun experience to throw out the 4oz size of my favorite leave-in hair conditioner and the container it was in. Airport security doesn't care if the bottle isn't full, they look at the size label on your item. If it's over 3 oz., you can kiss your favorite body care product, GOODBYE!

Take care of your liquids inside your checked luggage as they can easily explode. Cleaning up that mess isn't going to be what you want to do as the first vacation activity on your list. Make sure to place all liquids in a pressure-resistant container or double bag them in a Ziplock bag. Do not use a cheaper plastic bag, as they rip much easier. Check out Episode 26, Holiday Gift Guide for really great travel accessories.

You can also use a travel-ready toiletry bag that is clear. These are handy as the see-through travel cosmetic bags mean the agent can easily see what is in your bag and does not have to open and touch your cosmetics.

USE PACKING CUBES

When TSA thinks you have a suspicious object in your checked bag, you'll know because your bag will be jumbled and look like someone has just randomly searched through your suitcase and left a mess. In all actuality, that is precisely what happened. Second, you'll get what I call a "TSA Love Letter," a small black postcard-sized note saying that your bag was searched.

Then it dawned on me - they just searched my bag with all my personal, intimate clothing. They may have used gloves, but did they change their gloves between my bag and the previous bag that was searched? How do I know that their gloves were clean, that the bag they searched before me wasn't dirty, or that their dirty gloves just touched each of my single-serving food bags?

EEEEEEEEWWWWWWWWWWWWWWWWWW!

Since that time, I've used packing cubes in my suitcase. These neat little cubes come in an array of fashionable colors. They have zippers to compartmentalize the items in your luggage, including your food. I would definitely suggest getting a set of packing cubes. You can use makeup and jewelry organizers to give you more space for the rest of your food and your luggage.

Even though they are not see-through, packing cubes are a great way to keep searching hands off of your clothing and other items in your suitcase. If your luggage is chosen to be searched, the agent simply needs to open the cube to see what's inside, then zipper your cube closed.

Now, remember, this isn't a guarantee that the items you've packed won't be touched. I definitely can't vouch for another person's cleanliness. However, this packing method definitely decreases the chances of your personal items having germs from someone else's suitcase spread over them like mayonnaise on a sandwich.

FOR CARRY-ON BAGS

When packing food to bring with you on a carry-on, your best bet is to double Ziplock your food in plastic bags and place your food in an outside pocket of your carry-on bag. This will allow you easy access, as you will want to put your food in the clear plastic bag in a separate container on the scanner belt.

This will reduce suspicion that your food is a secret-weapon and may be used illegally. Additionally, this will help speed your way through security without having them dig through your bag and explain how your "I'm traveling with Celiac 101" speech.

FOR CHECKED LUGGAGE

Many times, I can get away with just a carry-on piece of luggage. However, there are some trips, like my two-week trip to Europe, where taking only a carry-on bag won't cut the space budget.

Remember the first paragraph about TSA going through my luggage? Looking around, I thought my things looked out of place, and then I found the card. Right after that, I noticed that my underwear and my food had been taken out and put back in a different spot.

Now you may be thinking, "well, they wear gloves," but they also handle other luggage, including another people's underwear, which may or may not be clean. They are even touching YOUR PACKED FOOD with their gloves, which may have been on other people's underwear: Yup, gross city!

In future trips, I've packed my food and my underwear in

plastic bags. Mind that your plastic bags have to be CLEAR or the TSA will open them and look through them.

Food items that are great to pack inside your luggage:

- ✓ Food bars that do not contain chocolate
- ✓ Crackers that are sturdy (not rice crackers) and will not break easily
- ✓ Protein in single-serve pouches
- ✓ Drink mix shaker (for your protein drink, see above!)
- ✓ Protein bars that do not contain chocolate
- ✓ Snack mixes that are sturdy (do not crumble easily) and do not contain chocolate
- ✓ Fruit leathers
- ✓ Nuts and nut mixes (without chocolate) sensitive or allergic to!
- ✓ Trail mix (no chocolate)
- ✓ Make sure to be a label reader for other ingredients (besides gluten) which you may be sensitive or allergic to!

HOW TO PACK YOUR FOOD

I use snack bag sized plastic bags, label them, and put my single servings inside the snack bag. I then take a gallon plastic bag and put my individual serve bags inside the big bag. Make sure to squeeze out any excess air to prevent your bags from exploding.

A website I found which sells travel-sized items is Minimus https://www.minimus.biz. They specialize in travel-sized items. A quick search in their search bar will give you a comprehensive list of the items that are tagged gluten-free. As always, double-check the ingredients list. When in doubt, check with the manufacturer. Check out Episode 26 for travel organizers you can use for food and great gifts for that gluten-free person.

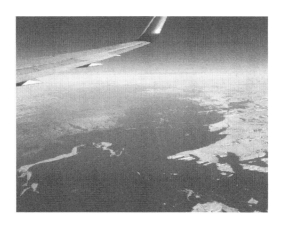

CALL THE AIRLINE DIRECTLY

To be safe, call ahead of time and ask the airline directly (not your travel agent) what gluten-free options they have on your specific flight. Have your flight confirmation number handy when you call the airline representative. Do not assume that all flights and airlines are created equal when it comes to food! Ask them what items they have available for snacks and how you can put in a special order for your meal.

Do this ASAP as airlines have different policies regarding the lead time on specialty diets. If you are dairy intolerant and gluten-free (as I am), you will have a hard time finding a meal that will cater to both. My suggestion is to always carry food with you in your carry-on and eat BEFORE you board the aircraft, if possible.

Below is a reference list of different airlines. Make sure to double-check and call ahead as information is continually changing because of supply chain issues with food. Airlines may have changed some of their policies.

Delta

https://www.delta.com/content/www/en_US/traveling-with-us/onboard-services/special-meals.html

"We offer a variety of meals, like vegetarian, diabetic, low-sodium and low-cholesterol meals to comply with special dietary requirements on flights that have scheduled meal service. Advanced notice is required. Not all special meals are available in all markets. At least 24 hours in advance, please request meals via 'My Trips - Special Service Requests 'or call 1-800-221-1212 to make arrangements for your special meal. Upon arrival at the departure gate, customers should advise the gate agent they have pre-ordered a special meal and also confirm with a flight attendant once onboard."

"Note the following exceptions apply: Special meal requests must be added for every new reservation. This information is not stored and is not automatically added to your reservation when you add your SkyMiles account. Be sure to select a meal from Delta's special meal listing as Delta does not fulfill meals that are not part of the special meal menu options. Special meals are not available on flights originating from ELP, ABQ, or TUS. Special meal offerings may vary depending upon regional catering availability. Kosher meals are not available on flights from CTG, LIM, UIO and BOG."

Alaska Airlines

https://www.alaskaair.com/content/travel-info/flight-experience/main-cabin/airbus-food-and-drink

"Now available on most flights where fresh food is available for purchase. You'll know if it's available for your flight if you see the "Food menu" option appear in your flight details within the Alaska Airlines mobile app, or when looking at your reservation on their site. Reserve food before flying ahead of time."

. . .

<u>Virgin America</u>

https://flywith.virginatlantic.com/gb/en/prepare-to-fly/dietary-requirements.html

"If you need a specific kind of meal, perhaps for medical or religious reasons, we have a range of specialized inflight meals we can serve you instead of our standard meals onboard."

"You will need to book your meal in advance. Simply log into 'My Booking' and you'll be given the option to book a specific meal. Order your meal more than 24 hours before your flight departs, and 48 hours if it's a Kosher meal. Special meal requests only apply to your main meal, and do not include the snacks and condiments we provide onboard. If you have special dietary requirements, we advise you to bring some snacks with you onto the flight."

<u>Virgin Atlantic</u>

https://flywith.virginatlantic.com/gb/en/prepare-to-fly/dietary-requirements.html

https://www.inflightfeed.com/virgin-atlantic/

"Make sure to order meals ahead of time that are listed as 'Does not contain gluten found in wheat, barley, rye, spelt, unripe spelt grain, oats kamut and triticale. This meal is suitable for passengers with coeliac disease or those passengers who have an intolerance to gluten.'"

"The following 16 special meals can be ordered on Virgin Atlantic services you will be required to give a minimum of 24 hours to order these options: Asian Vegetarian meal, Child meal, Fruit Platter, Gluten-free meal, Jain meal, Low-fat meal, Muslim meal, Vegetarian Lacto Ovo meal, Low Lactose, Baby meal, Diabetic meal, Hindu Meal, Kosher meal, Low salt meal, Vegan meal, Pureed meal." To book your meal or for further information, check with the airline.

ELIKQITIE

. . .

Jet Blue

https://www.cookinglight.com/healthy-living/travel/healthy-airline-food-options

JetBlue offers five special meals outside of their regular menu: vegan, a low-calorie meal, gluten-free options, "Plane Eats" for a kid's meal option or for those who have sensitive stomachs, and Kosher. Contact JetBlue's customer care line to indicate your dietary preference on your reservation or make a special note at the time of booking at least 24 hours ahead of the flight. Kosher meals must be requested a minimum of 48 hours in advance.

American

https://www.aa.com/i18n/travel-info/experience/dining/special-meals-and-nut-allergies.jsp

"Special meals to meet specific dietary, medical and religious needs are available on select flights. To make sure we can accommodate your needs, request your meal at least 24 hours before takeoff. Special meals are available in First or Business on most flights with meal service in the U.S."

"In addition, "Diabetic, Asian Vegetarian, Hindu, Muslim, Gluten Free, and Vegan meals will receive standardized and frozen pre-prepared meals, which will have a one year frozen shelf life."

Lufthansa

https://www.lufthansa.com/us/en/Special-meals

"Special meals can be ordered up to 24 hours before departure, provided that there is a confirmed booking in the required class. You have the option of ordering a special meal through your travel agency or online at My Bookings. There is no additional cost to you for this service. Please note that special meals are usually offered in Economy Class on flights of more than 185 minutes duration and in Business Class on flights of more than 75 minutes duration."

"Meal options for order include Diabetic, Gluten Free, Reduction Food, Low cholesterol, Low sodium, Lactose-Free, Vegetarian, Vegetarian Lacto-Ovo, Vegetarian Asian/Indian, Fruit Platter, Light Whole Food, Meat without fish, Child Meal, Kosher, Muslim and Hindu."

Spirit

https://customersupport.spirit.com/hc/en-us/articles/202097886-What-food-and-drinks-does-Spirit-offer-on-the-plane-

"We provide a variety of food and drinks that can be purchased using a debit or credit card. Cash is not accepted onboard because it's hard to make change in the sky. There is no complimentary beverage or snack service on Spirit flights. We do not offer any special dietary meals; however, our menu selection still provides a range of options that should meet most dietary requirements.

We cannot guarantee guests will not be exposed to peanuts during the flight and strongly encourage guests to take all necessary medical precautions to prepare for the possibility of exposure. In an effort to ensure your well being, please alert our gate agents and flight attendants if you do have an allergy, and we will create a peanut-free buffer-zone for you which includes the row you'll be seated in, the row in front of you, the row behind you and the corresponding rows on either side of the aisle as well."

. . .

UNITED

https://www.united.com/ual/en/us/fly/travel/inflight/dining/special.html

"We offer special meals on select routes when breakfast, lunch or dinner is scheduled. A special meal can be requested at the time of booking or by adding a request to an existing reservation. If special meals are available on a flight, you will be able to make a special meals request during the booking process after signing in to your MileagePlus account. MileagePlus account holders can also add special meal preferences to their profiles for use with bookings made through United.com. When signing in to your MileagePlus account and making a reservation on United.com, if you have a special meal preference set in your profile, you should verify that the correct special meal has been assigned to the applicable traveler's name prior to confirming the reservation.

If booking outside of United.com, a specific request must be made through the original booking channel for the available special meal to ensure it is included in the reservation, or by contacting the United Customer Contact Center."

QATAR AIR

https://www.qatarairways.com/en/services-special/special-meals.html

"Qatar Airways cannot guarantee an environment free from allergens (e.g. eliminating tree-nuts, peanuts, eggs, milk and other items that might cause an allergic reaction). Hence Qatar Airways regretfully does not accept responsibility for allergic reactions of any extent to the passengers. Passengers suffering from severe food allergies may consider a few precautions if they are concerned that they might be at risk of allergen exposure, such as: bringing their own meals and informing the airline or on-board crew of specific allergies."

"Qatar Airways does not provide nut-free meals. We regret the inconvenience, we do not guarantee against cross-contamination of nuts within our in-flight network. Passengers are requested to bring their own meals, which do not require chilling or re-heating. Please inform the cabin crew of your sensitivity or any allergen information and they will assist with any available meal options on board."

Emirate Airlines

https://www.emirates.com/us/english/before-you-fly/travel/dietary-requirements.aspx

"We serve gluten-free and lactose-free meals, as well as meals to suit other medical conditions. We can't guarantee our meals are nut-free. We serve nuts on all our flights, either as a meal ingredient or as an accompaniment to drinks. Other passengers may also bring food on board that contains nuts, and traces of nut residue could be passed on to other surfaces of the aircraft as well as through the air conditioning system. If you have a nut allergy, we recommend discussing your travel plans with your doctor before you fly. If you have a specific diet, you can choose from our range of special meals instead of from our onboard menu. Simply book a special meal up to 24 hours ahead of your flight through Manage Your Booking."

"Some of our special meals aren't available in Economy Class on flights lasting less than two hours. You won't need to book a child's meal or baby meal in advance unless they have a specific diet as we automatically identify children and infants within a booking. All meals are Halal certified."

PLAN AHEAD FOR YOUR FLIGHT

I always tell others who have food sensitivities to carry food with you on your carry-on. I was once upgraded to first class on a flight, which was an amazingly comfortable seat. Still, I couldn't eat any of the menu options they had available.

Carrying food on your flight with you prevents you from being without food. Make sure to take healthy options with you, as eating lots of sugar when you are on a plane isn't a good idea. Airports are generally lacking in food choices. If your connecting flight gets in late, you won't have the option of walking to another terminal to find different food. Carry enough food with you to get you to your destination.

❋ 13 ❋
GLUTEN FREE ROAD TRIPS

I really enjoy a great road trip. From an extended weekend to a planned multi-day trip, or multi-week adventure, road trip vacations can be as relaxed or fun-filled as you'd like! I love to stop and check out a small local museum or eat at places I've never heard of. You can make many detours with the freedom of a road trip that you cannot do with other types of travel.

Road trips are great as you can carry more of a variety of gluten-free goodies. I also love road trips as you can discover new markets and pick up food along the way to add to your gluten-free stash. Another reason road trips are super awesome is you don't have to worry about where you are going to eat. Just find a nearby park, pull over at a 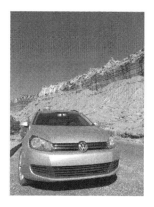 view area or rest stop, and have your very own gluten-free takeout spot to eat! You can find some stunning overlooks to stop and eat without the cost of expensive restaurant service.

During my years of eating gluten-free, I've found a few ways to lessen the hardship of gluten-free on the road. This is one of the easiest ways to travel, giving you the most dietary flexibility. Check out Episode 13 where I talk about gluten-free road trips.

PROS OF ROAD TRIPS

One of the excellent pros of a road trip is you will always have safe food to eat with you at all times! It's a good idea to pack about three to four days' worth of food when you take off for a trip lasting 7 days or more. You can easily use a search engine and GPS to locate food stores that carry gluten-free items. Also, use the resources mentioned in Chapters three and five to locate your favorite foods. Remember, if you are in a small town, you are less likely to find gluten-free food, unless you drive in California or Oregon, so plan accordingly! Best benefits when hitting the road are:

✓ Get to see places you wouldn't usually see in a plane, cruise or other scheduled trips

✓ Can stop anywhere you want to stop

✓ Economical

✓ Family-friendly, spend lots of time with your family/friends

✓ You choose your destinations and how long you want to stay

✓ Can add an extra destination along your route

✓ Very flexible time schedule can change itinerary along the way

✓ Amazing photo opportunities along your journey

✓ Can take breaks whenever you'd like

✓ Take gluten-free food with you, always have safe food to eat

✓ Discover new gluten-free foods along the way in the places you visit!

CONS OF ROAD TRIPS

✓ Have to make sure you have gas stations to stop at when driving in remote places

✓ The car must be reliable and inspected before you go on a road trip to ensure safety

✓ Towing can be an issue if your vehicle breaks down on a road trip

✓ Food safety can be an issue if you are in a small town and are eating out

WHAT FOODS SHOULD I TAKE ON A ROAD TRIP?

Some foods travel better than others on a road trip. Elements and variables, you will need to consider when taking food are:

- The number of gluten-free people on your road trip
- Season and time of year you are traveling
- Will the weather change significantly over the geographic region you are
- traveling on your trip?
- Will the non-gluten-free peeps coming on your trip eat your food?
- Do you want gluten-eaters eating your food?
- Does the food you're bringing need refrigeration when purchased or after
- the container of food is opened?

- Is the food sturdy (aka the food will not easily break apart, creating a mess

✓ Bottled water, vitamin water or other beverage which is low in sugar
✓ Trail mix without chocolate chips
✓ Peanuts, nut mix, trail mix. Always read the labeling and ingredients on trail mixes!
✓ Granola or protein bars that do not melt easily
✓ Single-serve ready to eat protein drinks
✓ Protein powder
✓ Fruits such as grapes, apples, and other fruits that are easy to transport
✓ Ready to eat, shelf-stable foods such as nut butter and hummus in single-serve packages
✓ Tuna and other meats in single-serve shelf-stable packaging
✓ Shelf-stable non-dairy kinds of milk
✓ Squeeze Packets of apple sauce and other fruit squeezes

ITEMS WHICH ARE NOT SO GREAT TO TAKE ON A ROAD TRIP:

✓ Chocolate or items that contain honey (all of these will melt, causing a big mess on your journey)
✓ Eggs
✓ Easily bruised fruits and vegetables such as tomatoes (which are really a fruit),
strawberries, raspberries
✓ If you do get a container of berries, make sure they are eaten within 24 hours to
avoid spoiling
✓ Watermelon
✓ Animal products that spoil easily such as dairy

STORING FOOD IN YOUR CAR

The interior of your car can easily reach 140 degrees during the summer! Remember to think about melting food and food spoilage in your vehicle. This can get super messy and a hassle to clean-up! You can also end up throwing out the food you can't eat because it's melted and too dirty to eat. Also, consider taking items packaged in cardboard or plastic food containers - do NOT bring along glass items as they can easily break.

Several companies make great travel food: 88 Acres, Deliciousness, KaPop!, Jai Mix, Vivian's Live Again, Mom's Gluten Free. You can order online directly from most companies on their website.

OVERSTOCKING FOOD ON YOUR ROAD TRIP

It's easy to buy a boatload of food and stash it in your car! Remember to keep only two to three days of food with you unless you have a cooler. Collapsible coolers are better to save space. If you want food to stay cold for an extended time, Yeti brand coolers are a great choice, and a bit more pricey, but the best option if you are not going to have an opportunity to stop for ice. Grab dry ice (not regular ice) as it lasts much longer. Be careful if you have small kiddos, you don't want to touch dry ice as it can burn you.

CARRY FOOD WITH YOU

Carry food with you at all times. This can be easy when you find out what you like and keep your favorite foods on hand. Always bring yummy snack foods with you for the ride. Gas Stations do not have many gluten-free offerings, except for Oregon and California. These are the only two states which I have found more than two or three safe snacks to eat at convenient stores.

For ultimate safety, only bring Certified Gluten-Free (look for the GF with the circle) or snacks that you have eaten at home and have found safe. Taking a chance with a new snack on-the-road, unless it's certified gluten-free, can be risky and create digestive havoc on your vacation!

Remember to not carry chocolate with you on your road trip, chocolate melts and makes a mess. Purchase chocolate on-the-go, so when you get a craving for the world's most perfect food, you can eat it, throw away the wrapper and not have to worry about the mess. Toss leftover chocolate because it's not worth the melted mess you have to clean up afterward.

Coconut is one of my favorite foods; however, when solid, coconut oil melts very quickly. Make sure to read the ingredients and eat any foods with coconut oil without storing leftovers.

🌿 14 🍂

CAMPING GLUTEN-FREE

Camping is a great adventure, and I really love living outdoors for several days. Sleeping outdoors creates a sense of understanding of nature when you sleep among the trees. I find this experience of sleeping close to the ground in a tent or in my hammock between two trees very grounding.

I also love having a campfire every night, not caring about smelling like campfire smoke or makeup. Truly unique memories are made when hiking beautiful trails, waking up to the sunshine beaming through your tent, and eating as many s'mores as humanly possible! There are so many things to love! Additionally, camping gives me a broader appreciation for running water and modern showers! After reading this chapter, check out Episodes #13, #86, #88 and #89 on gluten-free camping.

Few activities are a must when camping. You definitely will want to hike, rent a bike and ride on bike trails, and make at least one camping meal at night. Although I like to cook and bake at home, there's something about camping that creates a feeling of being OK

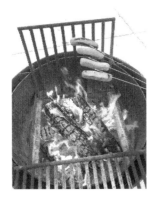

with throwing a bunch of food in one bowl and eating dinner. It's most likely that I'm super hungry from hiking all day.

If the park or place you are camping at offers nighttime sky programs, definitely give it a go! I'm a fan of astronomy and love planetariums and watching the night sky. If the spot you are camping doesn't offer a night program, check the area. You may be able to find a tourism business that provides stargazing.

PROS OF CAMPING:

✓ Get to be outdoors 24/7 and really immerse yourself in nature
✓ Have many hours of quality downtime with the people who are camping with you
✓ Biking, hiking and spotting animals are some of the many activities you can do outdoors
✓ Taking what you need with you - living minimally for a short time
✓ Very budget-friendly!
✓ Fun to meet other campers and many children for your kids to play with
✓ Eating meals cooked by the campfire
✓ SMORES - the main food group of camping

CONS OF CAMPING:

✓ Get to be outdoors 24/7 and immerse yourself in nature when she decides to downpour in the middle of the night

✓ Must drive to campsite or fly-in and rental car and equipment

✓ A tent can leak unexpectedly, or animals can eat the food you brought with

you to the campsite

✓ The grocery store may be far away - you may have to take a large amount of

food with you

✓ May not be many gas stations around, checking your gas gauge often

CAMPING FOOD SHORTCUTS

I wanted to share great gluten-free food prep tips for creating meals, camping snacks, prepared camping food that is gluten-free, and food storage when you're camping. Take steps to eliminate the hassle and expending energy on clean up when you're camping with these camping tips!

READY-TO-EAT MEALS

If you want to avoid cooking every night (like I do), your best bet is to grab freeze dried gluten-free camping food. Now, I know what you are thinking, camping food must taste bad. This is what I thought until my cousin introduced me to camping food! There are many varieties of camping food, and some brands are more gluten-free friendly than others. An excellent way to look at many different types of camping food is to check out your local camping store or visit an REI store or look online for camping foods. Make sure to note the number of servings for each pack. Some packs are two servings, some are four servings, and other camping food comes in a single-serving for those who are backpacking on their own.

How to prepare pre-packaged camping food:

1. Grab the food you want to eat
2. Boil water
3. Open the bag, being careful not to tear off the self-sealing top
4. Take out the "it's meant to keep the food dry" packet
5. Pour boiling water in the bag
6. Wait around 10-15 minutes (or more), depending on your meal. Make sure to

read directions thoroughly before cooking.

These are quick, easy, and tasty. You can even reseal the bag and save leftovers, although that can get messy if the bag explodes on you (yes, that has happened to me).

There are several brands that offer gluten-free friendly camping food - some of which are Certified Gluten Free! Try different dishes and see which ones you like the best. Make a fun easy-camping night by having a backyard campout eating a gluten-free camping food!

Backpacker's Pantry

Backpacker's Pantry freeze- dried meals that are yummy and gluten-free. These lightweight, freeze-dried, gluten-free meal packs are designed to be free of gluten. "From potato stew with beef to Santa Fe style rice and beans with chicken, there are plenty of delectable options for just about every type of appetite. You can even get gluten-free risotto with chicken, crafted to mimic the texture and flavor of the original Italian dish with a creamy blend of parmesan cheese, rice, broccoli, corn, onion, bell pepper and tomato."

Their website makes it easy to find gluten-free choices for breakfast, gluten-free lunch, or gluten-free dinners. You can also sort food by new gluten-free food items. For breakfast, try their carrot-cake pancakes with pineapple, raisins and coconut milk or their Summit Scramble complete with milk and peppers. These sound like an amazing breakfast or dinner after a long hike!

For dinner, try their Katmandu Curry, Pad Thai with Chicken, or Jamaican Style Rice Jerk with Beans. With over 60 different entrees to choose from, you are sure to find one that you can see yourself eating around a campfire!

Mountain House Adventure Meals

Certified gluten-free goodness leads the way with Mountain House Entrees. Chicken Teriyaki, Pad Thai with Chicken, and Yellow Curry Chicken and Rice to name a few of the choices. I like that these are certified gluten-free as we know that these are safe for Celiacs.

There are eight gluten-free breakfasts including Scrambled Eggs with Bacon, Spicy Southwest Breakfast Hash and Scrambled Eggs with Ham and Pepper.

Good To Go Meals

Are great as they give you many more gluten-free and vegetarian options. If you're vegetarian and gluten-free this is a good choice.

The company motto is to create the most delicious meals, using clean ingredients, to be enjoyed wherever your adventures take you. "Chef Jennifer's creations are thoughtfully crafted to provide a meal that not only tastes great but is truly good for you. Whether you've hiked all day for that summit view, rose with an alpine start to earn those backcountry turns, or are simply looking for an easy-to-make option at home, all you need is boiling water and in minutes you'll have a delicious meal." Gluten free choices cooked up by Chef Jennifer are Herbed Mushroom Risotto, Kale and White Bean Stew, and Classic Marinara with Pasta.

MARINATING GLUTEN FREE FOODS

An easy and efficient way to prepare your marinated food is to take your favorite gluten-free salad dressing and place your meal to be marinated into a double Ziploc. If you are using tofu, make sure to use firm tofu and plan to eat the first or second night, as tofu can fall apart quickly. Also, make sure to cut in thick slabs or cubes to reduce the change of your tofu becoming crumbles for your dinner.

For a quick and easy marinade, take your food to be marinated, and place it in a Ziploc bag. Add favorite salad dressing, just enough to coat your food. Place in double Ziploc, close bag, take all air out, then seal. Keep cool until ready to use.

BARBEQUING GLUTEN FREE

Make sure to scrub down the grill if you are using a park or campsite grill. Remember, you can't burn off the gluten protein from the grill, it has to be cleaned off. To be totally safe, it's best to put down heavy-duty aluminum foil before using the grill to create a clean barrier between your food and the grill.

Also, make sure not to use marshmallow sticks or skewers that have been used by someone eating regular wheat graham crackers. Mark gluten-free skewers with twist ties, colored ribbon, or colored masking or duct tape, so they are easily recognized when you go to use them again. Make sure when you are cleaning skewers that the gluten-free skewers are cleaned first, then the glutened skewers. These practices will avoid the chance for cross-contamination between the gluten eaters and you!

GLUTEN FREE CAMPING SOUPS AND CHILIS

To create easy soups, prep and blend your spices ahead of time and put them in an air-tight container. Label your container. Use dried spices instead of fresh if you are not going to use them in the first two days. Then, bring along canned items that you are going to use to make your soup. Make only the amount you need for one night - storing leftovers is time and energy-consuming.

GLUTEN FREE CAMPING AND HIKING SNACKS

If you are going hiking and need hiking snacks, the most efficient way to pack these is to buy single servings. Put one type of snack in each Ziploc bag - this is one of the expenses I will incur because Ziploc is sturdier than other brands of plastic storage bags.

For example, if you have 14 different flavors of squeezable fruits, put all the squeezable fruits in one Ziploc bag. When you are packing snacks for a hike, you can easily find which flavor you want. Give your kids several snacks they can choose from any of the snack bags you have brought. This is an easy way to distribute snacks before a hike.

You can also give each child a Ziploc with their name on the front with a permanent marker. This way, their bag is their responsibility, and they won't accidentally take someone else's snacks when it's time to stop and eat.

✓ Protein drinks are a great healthy and fast snack to eat when on the go

✓ Granola bars, such as KIND, are gluten-free and a tasty treat

✓ Applesauce and other fruit pouches are a great snack

✓ Tuna, salmon and other meats in aluminum pouches are easy to use when

hiking or camping

✓ Protein bars (as long as they aren't coated) are a tasty snack

✓ Crackers, nut butter (Jason's has nut butter in single-serving packets)

✓ Shelf-stable non-dairy kinds of milk in a single serving or quart size

✓ Avocados, apples and other fruits that store well without refrigeration

✓ Nuts

MY FAVORITE GLUTEN FREE HIKING SNACKS

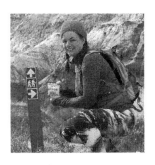

To reduce the time spent cleaning up and avoid messy foods when you pack for travel, you'll want to get as many single-serving packages as possible. Make sure not to bring snacks with a coating or a large amount of chocolate that can melt. Remember to try out food before you take a bunch with you on your vacation.

- NuGo With a variety of vegan, certified gluten free bars and cookies
- 88 Acres Seed butters and bars
- KaPop In different flavors including Siracha, 1oz and 3oz size

- Yes! Sesame based bars
- Justin's nut butters Single serving if you don't have a nut allergy person with you
- Orgain bars and protein drinks Blueberry almond bars and protein drinks in flavors
- Bobo's foods Stuffed oat bites
- Autumn's Gold Grain free granola bars
- Veggie Copia Pre-packaged olives and single serve hummus perfect for hikes!
- Mozaics Chips Great chips, come in single serving bags
- Handfulls Snacks Perfect alternative for regular trail mix, comes in delicious flavors
- Jai Mix a wonderful Eastern Indian blend of curry, nuts, coconut and other spices for an amazing trail mix

STORING FOOD WHEN CAMPING

Prepare just enough food for the group you are feeding. Storing extra food can be time-consuming and messy, especially if the container you are storing your food in breaks open! NEVER LEAVE FOOD OUTSIDE YOUR TENT, EVEN IF it is COLD! This can attract a variety of animals including bears that will not be gracious to you if you come in between them and their food!

STORING FOOD IN YOUR CAR

There are many ways to transport and store food when on the road or camping. I wish I had this information on my first camping trip. It would have saved me hours of prep and clean up time, giving me more time for adventure.

When I go on a road trip, I get shallow plastic boxes.

Why shallow? I can more easily organize my food and see my food because it's one layer deep and not several layers. If you get containers with a sunken top, you can easily tape a paper label to the bin to see what is in that container. Put canned, aluminum packaged, nut butter, snacks, and other sealed items in these bins.

NEVER leave open food in containers or your cooler, especially if you are in bear country. They can peel down a locked door car window to get to your food. Definitely NEVER store or bring any food, toiletries (because they smell like food to a bear), or any food wrappers into your tent. This will attract bears at night, and they don't like that you are preventing them from getting to their food.

Make sure to store your food in an animal-proof container, especially if you are in an area with bears! Bears can smell food for miles away, so don't think the bear won't come looking for a small amount of food inside your car.

Bears can peel back a car window (yes, actually peeled back like the window was a sticker) for a granola bar left inside their car!

Check to see if the campground you are going to provides an animal-proof container you can use for no extra charge. Many of the national parks offer animal-proof containers which you can use for your food.

Again, NEVER, EVER STORE FOOD INSIDE YOUR TENT OR IN YOUR CAR. The bears will come looking for it and find you and your camping friends sleeping next to the food!

ICE

Use dry ice! There are several reasons not to use regular ice in your cooler.

- Regular ice is heavier when you first get the ice and even heavier when the ice melts and you have a pool of water in your cooler
- Food in cooler gets wet when your ice melts
- Have to throw out good, expensive food - ever tried to eat wet gluten-free bread?
- Dry ice lasts much longer than regular ice.

Be careful not to touch dry ice with your hands as you can get a burn. Handle with paper or a towel! Although a bit more expensive, dry ice is worth the extra cost because of the benefits listed above.

If you can't get dry ice, buy a block of ice. While it can still melt in your cooler, a block of ice is easier to handle and fits neatly inside your cooler. Not every gas station or supermarket will carry ice blocks, but you can find block ice at KOA campground offices around the nation. You don't have to stay at a KOA to purchase items from their campground stores.

COOLERS

Best cooler: Yeti coolers, they are pretty pricey, starting at $79.99 for a lunchbox. However, they are the best option when you are not near any dry ice for days. The description from their website reads, "Extreme insulation power and durability are bare minimum requirements for every cooler we make — and we never stop there. Our hard coolers don't flinch in the face of snowstorms, the beating sun, or even bears, and our soft coolers are leakproof, waterproof, and quick to carry. As for our foldable lunch bag, that's only for those of you who enjoy ice-cold drinks and a fresh meal on your lunch menu."

ELIKQITIE

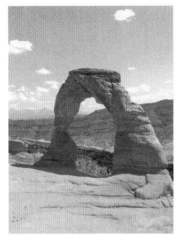 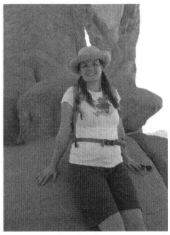

Hiking to Delicate Arch in Arches National Park is a popular hike in Moab, Utah

15
CRUISING GLUTEN FREE

Cruising is a great way to travel to several destinations in one trip. Food and non-alcoholic drinks are usually included in the price of the cruise. Once you board the ship, the only additional expenses you will incur are souvenirs, tipping, and alcohol.

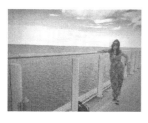

For many cruises, there are the regular dining options that are covered in the cost of your cruise and other restaurants, outside of regular dining rooms, that are not covered in the cost of your ticket. Some cruise lines are better than others when it comes to gluten-free dining. I travel Princess Cruise Lines as they have a dedicated kitchen space, a dedicated gluten-free chef and I've never been sick once on any of the several cruises I've taken with Princess.

Listen to Episode #40 "The 411 on Cruising" and Episode #41 "How to Cruise Gluten-Free" for more great information about cruising.

PROS OF CRUISING

✓ Visit multiple locations
  ✓ All food is included in the price of a cruise
  ✓ Many activities to do on the ship for all ages and interests
  ✓ Kids club where kids and teens can hang out and enjoy activities suited for their age group
  ✓ Safe for families and children
  ✓ Can do as much or as little as you want
  ✓ Excellent service from the staff
  ✓ Fantastic food, very good with making exceptions for food allergies/ sensitivities
  ✓ Meet other interesting people at your table during dining
  ✓ Your cabin moves with you - no need to worry about packing and unpacking multiple times

CONS OF CRUISING

✓ Have a limited amount of time at the port of call
  ✓ Not able to experience much of the culture of the area
  ✓ Limited activities due to time at port
  ✓ Do not get to choose where to stop
  ✓ Seasickness can make your trip, well, let's say, not good

BOOKING YOUR CRUISE

Book online through the cruise line or your favorite website or travel agent. To book luxury cruises, I would highly recommend Labbe Travel. They have a high level of service and are exceedingly amazing at finding one-of-a-kind getaways for your next adventure. Find them online at https://labbe-travel.com.

After booking your ticket, make sure to call the cruise line with your itinerary cruise number and tell them you are gluten-free. Generally, you want to go through your dietary restrictions about 90 days ahead of your departure date. If you book last minute, most cruise lines can still make accommodations, however; last minute details added to your account may not be in their system when you board the ship. When you make last minute reservations, make sure to check with your cruise associate that your diet restrictions are connected to your account.

Here is a list of popular cruise lines, in alphabetical order, with their contact information and the directions from their website that they suggest, when booking a cruise with their line. Please note: some cruises own multiple cruise lines, and although they have the same owner, their policies regarding specialty diets may differ. Always check with the specific cruise line you are traveling with on your vacation. You can also relay this information to your travel or booking agent who will make arrangements with the cruise line.

American Cruise Lines

https://www.americancruiselines.com/general-information/faqs

"American Cruise Lines will work to cater any dietary needs. Please tell your cruise specialist approximately two weeks prior to your cruise so that we may plan accordingly. Refrigeration is available to store insulin or other medications requiring protection."

Argyll Cruise (Scottish)

https://www.argyllcruising.com/life-on-board/example-menu/

"Before joining us aboard Splendour we ask each guest if they have any food allergies or special dietary requirements. We happily cater for vegetarian, vegan, gluten-free and many more. Please speak with Jamie about any special dietary requirements or allergies you may have. We want to make sure you have a memorable experience as you cruise the Scottish islands!"

Carnival

https://www.carnival.com/about-carnival/special-needs/dietary-needs.aspx

Carnival has gluten-free offerings such as gluten-free pizza dough, pasta, deli bread and hamburger buns, as well as frozen desserts and yogurt on hand, and gluten-free cake is available upon request a day or two ahead of time.

"Carnival can provide our guests with meals suited to the following special dietary needs: vegetarian, low-cholesterol, low-fat, low-carbohydrates, low-sugar, and gluten free. Our chefs will make every effort to fulfill your requests and will gladly prepare freshly-made options that meet your dietary needs. Once on board, we ask you to speak with the headwaiter or dining room host in advance, so they can assist in planning your daily meals in the dining room. This will allow us the necessary time to prepare foods, as requested, in a timely manner."

"Gluten-free pizza dough, pasta, bread for deli sandwiches, and hamburgers buns, as well as cake are available upon request. Plus, our frozen desserts and yogurt are gluten-free. All items are freshly prepared and may take a little longer than regular menu items. Gluten-free beer, Estrella Daura, is available for your enjoyment."

They also provide prepackaged kosher meals. If you're

requesting kosher meals, you must let us know two weeks advance of your cruise.

Celebrity

https://www.celebritycruises.com.au/life-on-board/onboard-facilities/restaurants-cafes/special-dietary-needs/

"Celebrity Cruises® is the first cruise line in the industry to introduce DineAware. The program provides set standards for food allergy and intolerance education throughout the food and beverage industry. All our restaurant and serving staff receive training through the DineAware program. Also, annual retraining is provided to ensure that we keep abreast of the latest information regarding the 14 major food allergens and intolerances. Our guests with special dietary needs can dine in confidence knowing that their food needs are top priority and will be readily accommodated while on board. Celebrity Cruises® is DineAware committed. We deliver excellent dining experiences for all guests to the best of our ability."

Crystal Cruise

http://www.crystalcruises.com/cruises/cruise-guidebook/before-you-sail-checklist/special-dietary-requests

"If you require a special diet, including any food allergies, or need specific food items during your cruise, we ask that you please submit your written dietary requests to our Onboard Guest Services Department by fax: 310-785-3975 or email: YachtButler@CrystalCruises.com at least 90 days (3 months) prior to sailing, and confirm your arrangements with the Food and Beverage staff on the day of embarkation. There may be a charge for some special requests, as well as any applicable shipping fees."

. . .

Disney Cruise

https://disneycruise.disney.go.com/guest-services/special-dietary-requests/

Although a bit on the pricey side, Disney is also known for its amazing service when accommodating dietary concerns. I've never been sick when eating a sit down meal at Disney and have always been impressed at the level of service and the amount of knowledge that Disney chefs contain in their head!

"By substituting different ingredients and approaches, Disney Cruise Line can accommodate the following common food allergies at our table-service restaurants:

- Gluten or wheat
- Eggs
- Fish
- Milk or lactose
- Peanuts and tree nuts
- Shellfish
- Soy
- Corn

"Additionally, lifestyle or cultural meal options, including Kosher and Halal, may be available upon advance request at no additional charge. Be sure to notify the Disney Cruise Line Contact Center or your travel agent of your request. Please note: These requests cannot be accommodated at our Quick Service locations or through in-room dining."

"For concerns regarding life-threatening or severe dietary allergies, notify the Special Services team at 407-566-3602 as soon as possible, prior to your cruise. Once aboard the ship, dietary allergies should also be brought to the attention of your Head Server."

. . .

Holland America

https://www.hollandamerica.com/blog/topics/food-beverage/special-dietary-needs-its-easy-to-cruise-with-holland-america-line/

"Travelers with Celiac disease or gluten sensitivities will find that items made without gluten are marked with the symbol of wheat next to their descriptions. If you are excited about a menu item, but not sure if it is gluten free or contains another allergen, speak to your server and our culinary team to be sure that each meal is safe and healthy for you to enjoy."

Norwegian Coastal Express

https://www.ncl.com/it/en/cruise-faq/dietary-needs

"If you have any food allergy or a dietary requirement that requires Kosher meals or gluten-free food products, please advise a Norwegian Reservations Agent, or your Travel Agent at the time of booking. Obtaining the product for many of these requests requires 30-days' notice prior to sailing, and we want to ensure that we are able to fulfil your request. We cannot guarantee Kosher Meal requests made within 30 days of sail date."

"Our travelers with Celiac disease or gluten sensitivities will find items made without gluten are marked with the symbol of wheat next to their descriptions. Our Dive-In burgers also can be made with gluten-free buns. While our main ingredients are listed with each menu item, you may not know if a meal contains trace amounts of other common allergens such as nuts, milk or butter. If you are excited about a menu item, but not sure if it is gluten free or contains another allergen, speak to your server and our culinary team to be sure that each meal is safe and healthy for you to enjoy."

. . .

Oceania Cruises

https://www.oceaniacruises.com/experience/dining/

"Vegetarian, Kosher and special diets upon request Please request 90 days prior to voyage."

Pearl Seas Cruises

https://www.pearlseascruises.com/frequently-asked-questions

"Pearl Seas Cruises will work to cater any dietary needs. Please tell your cruise specialist approximately two weeks prior to your cruise so that we may plan accordingly. Refrigeration is available to store insulin or other medications requiring protection."

Princess Cruise Line

https://www.princess.com/learn/faq_answer/onboard/dining_nightlife.jsp

My favorite cruise line, on Princess, they have a gluten-free kitchen in which they create their gluten-free bread and desserts. Their bread is made on the ship, is very fresh and fluffy. One cruise my husband and I ended up sitting with a pair of sisters - one of which was Celiac - and we shared almost a half-loaf of bread every night at dinner together! Eating that delicious, fluffy and mouth-watering bread every night was such a treat.

Princess delivers for the gluten-free community as they do not add any gluten-laden flours to their soups, sauces or salad dressings! There are some meat dishes that have gluten, however; for the most part, many of their dishes are gluten-free. I have always received excellent service on this line, which is why I cruise with Princess when I travel.

"You or your travel consultant must advise Princess in

writing of any special diet, allergies or medical needs. Requests must be received no later than 35 days prior to departure for cruises to Alaska, Canada/New England, Caribbean, Hawaii, Mexico, Panama Canal and Coastal Getaways. For all other cruises, requests must be received no later than 65 days prior to departure. Once onboard, please check with the Maître D' to confirm your request."

"Any special dining requests (name brands, daily food order requests, sample menus, etc.) not related to medical or allergy requirements should be directed to the onboard dining staff and are not handled by our Dietary Office."

Royal Caribbean

https://www.royalcaribbean.com/faq/questions/dining-dietary-restrictions-customer-care

Royal Caribbean is another mainstream line with an excellent system in place for gluten-free cruisers; gluten-free sandwiches and pastries are always available in coffee shops; the buffet always has a marked gluten-free dessert on offer; Sorrento's has a separate oven for making gluten-free pizza; and all menus have gluten-free items marked, as well as a guide to inform diners which items have gluten.

"We make every effort to accommodate our guests' dietary requirements whenever possible. We can accommodate dietary needs such as: Food allergies, Gluten-free, Kosher, Low-fat, and Low-sodium. A variety of vegetarian Meals are available on all menus in the Main Dining Room and Windjammer Cafe every day. Guests do not need to make a special request for these meals."

"Lactose-free/soymilk, ensure, and kosher meals are available at no extra charge. All you have to do is notify us at least 45 days prior to sailing (90 days for European/South American Itineraries). Vegan menus are available upon request at the Main Dining Room. Kosher for Passover meal requests MUST be received 90 days in advance in order to be accommodated. Contact your travel advisor or Certified Vacation Planner and request that the remark be noted in your reservation details. If you made your reservation online at royalcaribbean.com you may add your request to the 'update personal information' section. You may also send an email request to special_needs@rccl.com; please include in the email the guests' names, booking number, ship name and sail date. E-mails will receive an automated response."

VIKING CRUISES

https://www.vikingrivercruises.com/frequently-asked-questions.html

"Every meal has vegetarian options on the menu, and our chefs are able to prepare low-salt or gluten-free cuisine. Guests requiring special diets such as diabetic or low-cholesterol meals must alert Viking Cruises one month prior to departure and inform the Maître d' when on board. The chefs will make every effort to accommodate these requests."

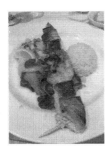 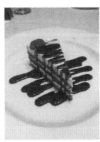 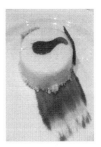

CHOOSING YOUR DINING ROOM

Now that you've decided on what cruise line you are going to travel; you must choose one dining room to eat in for dinner.

This may sound boring if you've never been on a cruise, but believe me, I've been on multiple cruises and have never been disappointed by the food that has been served to me, except for one cruise line.

Usually, the ship has several dining rooms that serve the same menu, which is included in the cost of your ticket. There are other dining rooms that are paid for service, however; the quality of the food at the "regular dining" is excellent. I would not eat at a paid for service restaurant for three reasons: 1. The person serving you isn't familiar with your food sensitivities, allergies and 2. They are going to have way fewer choices for you to eat 3. They are more likely to make a mistake when serving you food.

Choose one dining room you would like to eat for the rest of the week. Make sure to meet your maître D before the cruise starts and explain your food sensitivity/allergy/ Celiac with them ahead of time. Be clear with your maître D that you will be dining in that room all week for dinner.

PRE-ORDER YOUR FOOD THE NIGHT BEFORE

Now that you have established your dining room and met your maître D ask about pre-ordering your food for the next night. Choose what you want to eat and ask if it can be modified to be gluten-free. Review and check your order with the maître D or the head chef to make sure they have the correct order before they walk away.

Another thing you should know about cruising is when you order your food, you can order more than one item on their regular menu without an additional charge. For example, I remember once I had the option of a cold pear soup. After eating the cold pear soup, I was hooked! I asked for another pear soup and they brought one out. When cruising, you're on an unlimited gluten-free buffet! I never feel deprived or hungry on the cruise - I feel quite the opposite. When cruising, I know I have to work out every day if I want to keep my weight gain to three pounds for the week.

EATING AT YOUR SHIP'S DINING ROOM

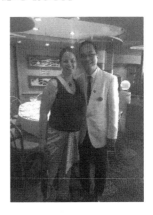

Let your waiter know you have a pre-order because of a food allergy as they may not understand Celiac Disease and explain to them that this is NOT a preference. Feel free to tell the maître d you put in your pre-order the night before and that you have a food allergy/sensitivity. Your food should come out with the rest of the food at your table, if not, let your maître d know that your food came out late.

THE BUFFET

Located on the top level of the ship. Look around to see what choices you can see are obviously gluten-free (fruit, salad without dressing). Ask for the head chef. The head chef will give you a tour of the buffet and let you know what foods are safe to eat. They are very knowledgeable about all the ingredients in the menu on the ship. Don't feel that you are bothering them by asking them every day what foods are safe to eat. Cruises are very service oriented! Be sure to mention the chef's name in your survey at the end of the cruise.

OTHER FOOD AROUND THE SHIP

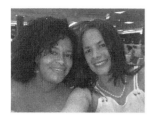

Some food may be labeled gluten-free, if it isn't, ask the waiter/waitress. You can also ask any maître D' on the vessel about the food or a chef. Sometimes the people serving the menu are not sure. Ask your server at dinner or breakfast if you want to eat a particular food, but not sure about its safety.

FOOD OFF THE SHIP

The food you are eating at port when you get off the boat can be risky. There are several resources you can use to find safe food. Use the tools laid out in Chapter 3 to navigate safe food on the shoreline!

SHORE EXCURSIONS

If you've never cruised before, a shore excursion is an activity you participate in when you are at a port. Cruise lines offer more pricey shore excursions. The benefit of purchasing a shore excursion through a cruise line guarantees that the ship won't leave without you.

Yes, that is correct. If you are out at port and don't get back to the ship before it leaves, the ship goes without you, and you are responsible for transportation to the next port your ship is docking. I have never had this happen to me as I always reserve shore excursions with at least two hours of buffer time. Also, the tour guide who is leading your excursion will usually ask you what cruise line you are on and when the ship leaves to get you back in enough time to get on board the ship. Many of the local tour guides are small businesses and give excellent tours to visitors.

I usually book through TripAdvisor or one of the popular online trip planners. You can participate in your choice of recreational activity that is suited to your adventure level. Walking, biking, historical, and e-bike tours are popular forms of entertainment. Snorkeling, scuba diving, and paragliding are sought-after water activities. Additionally, there are many different types of food and wine tours, depending on your cruise location.

I would not go on a food and wine tour as you are stuck with the restaurant that the tour is going to and do not choose where to eat. Yes, you could bring your own food, but sitting there. At the same time, everyone else has delightful culinary experiences while eating a granola bar really isn't a part of a relaxing vacation!

Also, avoid trips that offer lunch or dinner included, such as evening dinner cruises. Unless the dinner cruise specifically states they cater to allergies, they are a big no-no. With fixed menus and prepared food off-site, there isn't room for substitution, and you have no idea how the food was primed when created. Definitely do not participate in shore excursions that include food. There is a high risk to your health, and you won't have fun watching everyone else eat in front of you.

THE GUIDE TO TRAVELING GLUTEN FREE

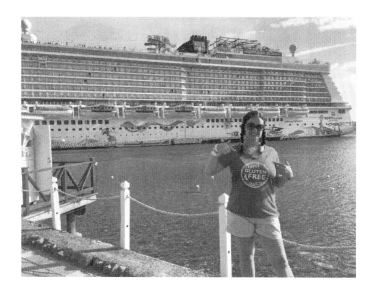

16

TOP TEN GLUTEN FREE FRIENDLY CITIES IN AMERICA

Isn't it frustrating when you travel for vacation only to find there are minimal options for you to eat? Does your level of anxiety go through the roof when you find yourself in a situation where you can't safely eat at restaurants nearby? Do you find yourself having to eat a snack you brought while everyone else enjoys "real" food?

One of the deciding factors for the location I'm traveling to is the availability of safe, gluten-free, Celiac-friendly food. So what elements of a city lend that town to being gluten-free friendly? While there isn't a "written in stone" order or process to find out which cities are more accommodating to our gluten-free community, cities that have the following characteristics usually have a better variety of safe food to eat for specialty diets such as Celiac:

- College towns
- Cities that value culture and art
- Locations that are highly densely populated
- Coastal towns

- Anywhere in California
- Cities that are older than 150 years

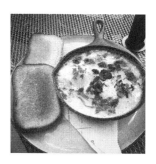

DEDICATED GLUTEN FREE AND GLUTEN-FREE FRIENDLY - WHAT'S THE DIFFERENCE?

Gluten-Free Friendly or Celiac-Friendly Restaurants

A gluten-free friendly or Celiac-friendly restaurant is a restaurant that offers gluten-free foods and is safe for Celiacs to eat at. This does not mean that no one has ever been sick at this establishment. What it does mean is that you have a high probability of finding several menu choices at a restaurant that is accommodating to those of us who live gluten-free.

Some features or extras a Gluten-Free friendly establishment may have:

- Tag your order gluten-free or allergy
- Put a label in the gluten-free food
- Dedicated prep space for gluten-free in kitchen
- Dedicated gluten-free kitchen space
- Dedicated fryer - only fry gluten-free items
- Gluten-free bread
- Gluten-free menu
- Choice of gluten-free desserts

Note that a gluten-free friendly restaurant's offerings depend on the head chef as they choose the menu. Chefs that are Celiac will have a great menu with excellent cuisine options! And it's always a big score to find a restaurant with gluten-free bread. Check with your server and have them check with the head chef to let you know which menu options they have that are safe for you to eat.

DEDICATED GLUTEN-FREE RESTAURANTS

A dedicated gluten-free restaurant is an establishment that is entirely free of gluten! When you get the menu, you can order anything you want off the menu, which is pretty exciting and is the best sense of normalcy when you are Celiac. When you find one of these gems, support this business! As a community, we need to make sure that these establishments know we appreciate the extra mile they go to feed us safe food and give us the ability to enjoy eating out like "normal" people!

Remember to use available technology, and reference Chapter 03 for tools you can use to see available gluten-free friendly and dedicated gluten-free options that are available to you when you travel. Also note, that there may be some restaurants on the app that are closed, and other new restaurants that have opened which are gluten-free friendly that are not yet listed on these platforms. Additionally, you may find a restaurant that isn't listed on any platform as being gluten-free friendly. Make sure to list the restaurant or request the establishment to be listed so others will know about it and have the opportunity to support a Celiac-friendly restaurant!

Below is a list of cities in America that have made my list for the top gluten-free friendly towns. This does not mean that these are the only towns that offer gluten-free food. However, these are the towns you will be able to eat comfortably with a variety of safe gluten-free restaurant choices as these towns have many dedicated and gluten-free friendly options available. This chapter lists a few of my personal favorites in each city. Additionally, you will be able to find more dedicated and gluten-free friendly restaurant options when searching more extensively using the apps mentioned in Chapter 03. Always make sure to call ahead to verify restaurant offerings and locations.

In addition to the dedicated gluten-free and Celiac-friendly restaurants on this list, you'll also find a link to the city's official visitor's guide, which has extensive information on fun activities and adventures you can do while visiting. Cities are listed in alphabetical order for ease of reference.

AUSTIN, TEXAS

Austin is known for its nightlife and music scene, but did you also know that you can find amazing gluten-free food as well? Check out the myriad of art, music, and activities you can do while visiting in Austin on their city website https://www.austintexas.org

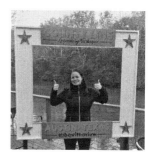

Gluten-Free Friendly

Max's Wine Dive, 207 San Jacinto Blvd, Austin, TX 78701 (512) 904-0111

This is the first place I go when eating out in Austin. Their gluten free fried chicken on top of a heaping stack of mashed potatoes are to die for! Perfectly seasoned chicken, pair this with a glass of white wine for the perfect gluten-free dish!

. . .

G'Raj Mahal, 73 Rainey St, Austin, TX 78701 (512) 480-2255

Best Indian food I've ever eaten in the States. Much of the menu is gluten free and they even have safe dessert choices.

Galaxy Cafe, 1000 W Lynn St, Austin, TX 78703 (512) 478-3434

Separate GF menu and tag "allergy" on your order. No separate kitchen space but use a separate toaster for gluten free bread. Great food and plenty of options.

Dedicated Gluten Free

ATX Cocina, 110 San Antonio St, Austin, TX 78701 (512) 263-2322

A 100% gluten-free Mexican restaurant serving quesadillas and tasty spicy salsa. Try their fish dishes and brussels sprouts.

Wilder Wood Restaurant and Bar, 1300 E 7th St, Austin, TX 78702 (512) 628-0184

Known for their burgers and carrot cake. Check out the buffet on Sunday as we have few chances to eat safely at a buffet!

Picnik 4801 Burnet Rd, Austin, TX 78756 (737) 226-0644

Accommodating staff. Definitely get the salted caramel banana pancakes, the everything bagel toast, the french toast, and the chicken tenders.

BOSTON, MASSACHUSETTS

One of the oldest cities in America, you'll find a rich American history walking through the streets of Boston and visiting the museums and places within our National Park Service. Save 45% on attractions to passes in the city at Visit Boston https://bit.ly/3gcb74E

Dedicated Gluten Free

Back Deck 2 West Street, Boston, MA 021112 (617) 670-0320

Dedicated kitchen space and fryer with many options. Order the Nonna burger or choose from a variety of items on their gluten-free menu. Dedicated fryer for yummy fried food!

Grainmaker 91 Summer St, Boston, MA 02110 (617) 482-0131

Order the Miso soup! They also serve a variety of delicious homemade beverages. Bonus: this place is dairy-free as well with amazing food and wonderful atmosphere.

Jennifer Lee's Gourmet Bakery 100 Hanover St, Boston, MA 02108 (978) 675-5116

From gluten-free Paninis to a variety of desserts, you can't go wrong with anything you order from Jennifer's.

Paris Creperie 278 Harvard Street, Brookline, MA 02446 (617) 232-1770

Many delicious French foods! Try their savory crepes, sweet crepes, and the Nutella hot chocolate. Staff is knowledgeable and aware of food allergies and will make sure your food is Celiac safe.

**Violette Gluten Free Bakery 1786 Massachusetts Ave, Cambridge, MA 02140
(857) 500-2748**

Great options for gluten-free, dairy free and vegan as well. Highly recommend the cupcakes, sourdough loaf, rosemary pita crackers, macarons and donuts!

CHICAGO, ILLINOIS

I can't begin to express the number of Celiacs in our community who have raved about eating in Chicago! Stay at the Magnificent Mile across the waterfront to experience the best views Chicago has to offer https://bit.ly/2OUHYzh

GLUTEN-FREE FRIENDLY

CHICAGO'S PIZZA 3114 N Lincoln Ave, Chicago, IL 60657 (773) 477-2777

If you're looking for deep dish pizza, you've found the right place! Although not dedicated gluten-free, they know how to treat their non-gluten clients with fresh bread and amazing gluten-free pizza.

DO-RITE DONUTS 50 W. RANDOLPH, Chicago, IL 60601 (312) 488-2483

Several gluten-free doughnut choices such as cinnamon sugar, chocolate frosted, and sprinkle frosted. Buy one, a half or dozen and bring these delicious, fluffy and tasty treats home in your suitcase! Call ahead to order in quantity so they can prep and clean for your order.

Flip Crepes 131 North Clinton Street, Chicago, IL 60661 (773) 321-0210

It's hard to find a good gluten-free crepe. The only other one I've found is in Seattle at Pike's Place Market. Definitely get a few savory and sweet crepes and split it with friends and family then buy as many mixes that you can stuff into your suitcase for your trip home!

DEDICATED GLUTEN FREE

BRIGHTWOK KITCHEN, 21 E Adams St, and 631 N State St., Chicago, (312) 583-0729

Gluten-free, dairy-free and peanut-free! Stir fry, potato fritters and great kids' meals. Get a build your own bowl option and bring the family for a bite to eat.

LITTLE BEET TABLE 845 N State St #101, Chicago, IL 60610 (312) 549-8600

Delicious gluten-free food with many dairy free and vegan options.

MINNEAPOLIS, MINNESOTA

In Episode #36, Kari from The Savory Celiac talks about gluten-free life in Minnesota. Listen to this episode to hear

Kari's favorite local spots to eat and check out what you can do to visit Minneapolis on their tourism website at https://bit.ly/30GQ9oc.

Gluten-Free Friendly

Red Cow 208 N 1st Ave, Minneapolis, MN 55401 (612) 238-0050
Terrific gluten free burgers, with Udi buns to pair with gluten free beer or cider. Clearly marked menu, dedicated fryer and amazing service.

Dedicated Gluten Free

Colita 5400 Penn Ave S, Minneapolis, MN 55419 (612) 886-1606
Exceptional food including the shrimp tempura tacos, fried green tomato salad, black bean hummus guacamole and churros! Wonderful atmosphere and service.

Burning Brothers Brewing 1750 W Thomas Ave, St Paul, MN 55104 (651) 444-8882 Excellent root beer and great gluten free food.

Sassy Spoon 5011 S 34th Ave, Minneapolis, MN 55417 (612) 886-1793
Food is great no matter what you order off the menu!

. . .

SIFT GLUTEN FREE 4557 Bloomington Ave, Minneapolis, MN 55407 (612) 503-5300

Tasty treats definitely take home the cookie dough. Super friendly staff and great gluten-free service.

NEW YORK, NEW YORK

New York is hard to beat when you're looking for gluten-free food, especially when it comes to the best gluten-free bakeries. Make sure to take an extra bag with you to bring home a variety of baked goods. Definitely check out Modern Bread and Bagel and get a bag of the most delicious gluten-free bagels in the States. Find culture, music, and history with your unforgettable visit to New York https://www.nyc.com/visitor_guide/

DEDICATED GLUTEN FREE

POSH POP BAKESHOP 192 Bleecker St, New York, NY 10012 (212) 674-7674

Favorites are the milk and cookies cake, chocolate chip cookie sandwich, Nutella s'mores brownie, and cinnamon roll. Bring your friends as they won't be able to tell it's gluten-free.

ROLLN 38 E 23RD ST, New York, NY 10010 (646) 869-0826

The only thing harder to find than great gluten free fried chicken is a dedicated gluten free sushi restaurant! Find out what it's like to eat amazing sushi when you don't have to worry about food safety.

. . .

ERIN MCKENNA'S BAKERY NYC 248 BROOME ST, New York, NY 10002 (212) 677-5047

Overwhelming amount of choices! In several cities around the US including Orlando at Disney Springs, Erin McKenna's is one of my favorite gluten-free bakeries.

RISOTTERIA MELOTTI 309 E 5th St, New York, NY 10003 (646) 755-8939

Great service, amazing and definitely leave room for dessert!

SENZA GLUTEN 206 SULLIVAN ST, New York, NY 10012 (212) 475-7775

Delicious and amazing food! Can't go wrong ordering any item from this menu.

INDAY 1133 BROADWAY, New York, NY 10010 (917) 521-5012

Amazing Indian food for lunch or dinner along with good service.

Little Beet Table 333 Park Ave S, New York, NY 10010 (212) 466-3330

Excellent service! Definitely try the NY strip steak, grass fed burger, mushroom and black bean burger. A variety of vegan and vegetarian options.

. . .

MODERN BREAD AND BAGEL 472 COLUMBUS AVE, New York, NY 10024
(646) 775-2985

Order bagels, breads, and pastries online and have them shipped right to your door. Best gluten free bagels.

FRIEDMAN 228 W 47TH ST, and 132 W 31st St, New York, NY 10036, (646) 876-1232

As good as the others around the city. Got the Friedmans burger with the GF bun and herb fries. Will probably check out the pastrami next time.

PHILADELPHIA, PENNSYLVANIA

Philadelphia has so many fun activities to see and do! From the many historical places to visit, the Philadelphia Zoo, and nightlife on South Street, you'll never run out of fun places to see! Check out Episode #67 to find out my favorite activities in my hometown of Philadelphia. Find out in Episode #65 about Michael from Gluten-Free Philly and his personal favorite gluten-free recommendations. Find out more about the "City of Brotherly and Sisterly Love" https://www.visitphilly.com

GLUTEN-FREE READING TERMINAL Market

Reading Terminal Market. RTM is an authentic Philly experience and offers a variety of dishes that are not only gluten-free, but the eating establishments are also from many different food cultures, which I love! When you're there, definitely check out Fox & Son. The owner, Rebecca, created a dedicated gluten-free restaurant that features such delicacies as funnel cake, fried Oreos, gluten-free corn dogs, and white birch beer. Birch beer is a northeastern beverage, similar to root beer, 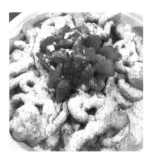 but on a more mouth-awakening level. Listen in on Episode #66 for my interview with Rebecca from Fox & Son about how she created my favorite dedicated gluten-free restaurant.

GLUTEN-FREE SOFT PRETZELS at the Italian Market in Philadelphia

IF YOU'RE IN PHILLY, definitely stop by the Italian Market on 9th street in Philadelphia. There are fabulous gluten-free finds at the market, including traditional Philadelphia foods such as gluten-free soft pretzels at Taffets, who also carry a variety of gluten-free baked goods such as baguettes.

DEDICATED GLUTEN FREE

SOUTHHOUSE 2535 S 13TH ST, Philadelphia, PA 19148 (267) 457-3682
Knowledgeable staff and great food!

ORIGINAL 13 CIDERWORKS 1526 N American St, Philadelphia, PA 19122 (215) 765-7000

Grab a glass of cider and have fun with the wall of board games.

Taffets Bakery & Store 1024 S 9th St, Philadelphia, PA 19147 (215) 551-5511

Grab gluten free soft pretzels Philly style at this small bakery shop. Also try their brownies!

Farmer's Keep 10 S 20th St, Philadelphia, PA 19103 (215) 309-2928

Healthy and tasty gluten free options for all.

Fox & Son Fancy Corndogs 51 N 12th St, Philadelphia, PA 19107 (215) 372-7935

Only place on Earth I know of where you can purchase a safe funnel cake! Also try the white birch beer and listen in on Episode #66 where I interview Rebecca, owner of Fox & Son.

Real Food Eatery 207 S 16th St, Philadelphia, PA 19102 (215) 608-8941

Create your own gluten-free bowl, absolutely delicious!

PORTLAND, OREGON

From museums to botanical gardens and historical places, Portland has various attractions to see and do! Check out Episode #10 as I interview Jason Elmore, founder of the Find Me Gluten Free App, as he talks about his favorite local restaurants. Visit their travel destination website to plan your next visit https://bit.ly/2CEsZHe

Dedicated Gluten Free

Schilling Cider House Portland 930 SE 10th Ave, Portland, OR 97214 (360) 608-8331
For the best selection of gluten-free brews in Portland, Schilling is the place to eat and drink.

Prasad 925 NW Davis St, Portland, OR 97209 (503) 224-3993
One of the most visited gluten-free places in Portland, this cafe is also dairy free with vegan options.

Kyra's Bake Shop 599 A Avenue, Lake Oswego, OR 97034 (503) 212-2979
Cinnamon rolls to wedding cakes, also offers dairy free and vegan options as well!

Gluten Free Gem Bakery140 NE Broadway St, Portland, OR 97232 (503) 288-1508
Definitely try the doughnuts, lemon poppyseed pound cake and quiche!

Butterfly Belly Asian Cuisine 323 NW Park Ave, Portland, OR 97209 (503) 788-7327

It's hard to find a good dedicated Asian restaurant, however; this Vietnamese restaurant is completely gluten and dairy free.

GroundBreaker Gastropub 2030 SE 7th Ave, Portland, OR 97214 (503)928-4195

Another option for safe fried food, definitely check out the buttermilk fried chicken bowl.

Petunia's Pies & Pastries 610 SW 12th Ave, Portland, OR 97205 (503) 841-5961

How can you go wrong with Pumpkin waffles? Definitely visit and bring home some of these wonderful, tasty and safe treats!

SAN DIEGO, CALIFORNIA

While many California towns offer gluten-free fare, I wanted to pick out my favorite place to go in California when I want to see museums and take in the culture. Visit Balboa Park and grab their multi-day pass to explore the many diverse museums in the beautiful, sunny California weather. Go to the San Diego Zoo to learn about our world's animals and definitely hang out with the Orangutans. https://www.sandiego.org/plan/visitors-information-services.aspx

Gluten-Free Friendly

. . .

LAS HADAS BAR AND GRILL 558 FOURTH AVE, San Diego, CA 92101 (619) 232-1720

Manager will come and talk to you about options, which are many. Dedicated kitchen space, they create delicious food and the wait staff are super helpful!

Cueva Bar 2123 Adams Ave, San Diego, CA 92116 (619) 269-6612

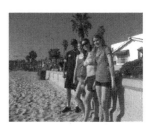

The staff was super knowledgeable about food restrictions with Celiac and will review food options. Separate kitchen for gluten free prep.

DUCK FOOT BREWING CO. 550 Park Blvd, San Diego, CA 92101(619) 550-1970

Dedicated kitchen space and great gluten free beer.

DEDICATED GLUTEN FREE

THE GLUTEN FREE BAKING CO 4594 30TH ST, San Diego, CA 92116 (858) 270-9863

Stop in for one or more of their delicious baked goods to go.

HEALTHY CREATIONS 376 N El Camino Real, Encinitas, CA 92024 (760) 479-0500

Grab one of their healthy menu items, including the popular panini.

. . .

Nectarine Grove 948 N Coast Hwy 101, Encinitas, CA 92024 (760) 944-4525

Many healthy breakfast and brunch options that are also dairy free!

Starry Lane Bakery 3925 Fourth Ave, San Diego, CA 92103 (619) 328-0500

Cinnamon rolls, brownies, and lemon raspberry tortes are among the many delicious options in this amazing bakery.

SEATTLE, WASHINGTON

A city of art and culture, this is the perfect destination for travelers who love food and art. When in Seattle, definitely take a day and visit Pikes Peak Market, where you'll find local 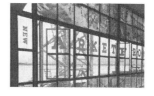 handicrafts, fresh seafood, and gourmet foods. While you're there, check out Crepe de France for delicious gluten-free crepes! Also, check out the Space Needle, and my favorite art museum Chihuly Garden and Glass See a list of Seattle's art and cultural attractions here https://bit.ly/3hEWt6G

Gluten-Free Friendly

Capitol Cider 818 E Pike St, Seattle, WA 98122 (206) 397-356

Safe use of beer taps for gluten-free beer and a dedicated gluten free kitchen!

Bamboo Sushi 2675 NE University Village Lane, Seattle, WA 98105 (206) 556-3449 Nice to Many gluten-free choices, servers are helpful and the menu also contains dairy free choices.

Casa Guadalajara 4105 Taylor St, San Diego, CA 92110 (619) 295-5111
Extensive gluten free menu with amazing Mexican food.

Lola 2000 4th Ave, Seattle, WA 98121 (206) 441-1430
Perfect stop for a Celiac friendly late night bite.

Cinnamon Works 1536 Pike Pl, Seattle, WA 98101(206) 583-0085
Definitely stop by this amazing bakery for the best gluten free cinnamon rolls.

Dedicated Gluten Free

Flying Apron 3510 Fremont Ave N, Seattle, WA 98103 (206) 442-1115
In addition to gluten-free all items are also vegan! Grab a baked good to go if you can't fit one in after eating lunch.

· · ·

Ghostfish Brewing Company 2942 1st Avenue South, Seattle, WA 98134
(206) 397-3898
Delicious food, great staff. I've had brunch and dinner here and everything has been great.

Nuflours 518 15th Ave E, Seattle, WA 98112 (206) 395-4623
Grab a coffee and a yummy baked treat from a bakery that is owned by another Celiac.

Razzis Pizzeria 1314 Howell St, Seattle, WA 98101 (206) 588-2425
Serving my favorite Italian food, the calzone! Definitely get a glass of wine or a gluten free cider along with your Italian fare.

WASHINGTON, DC, VIRGINIA

Visit DC to see America's second national capital behind Philadelphia. Definitely check out the historical monuments, see a show at the John F. Kennedy Center for the Performing Arts and view hundreds of works of art at the National Gallery of Art https://bit.ly/302uwjc

Gluten Free-Friendly

. . .

Legal Sea Foods 704 7th Street. N.W., Washington, DC 20001 (202) 347-0007

So many people from the gluten-free community rave about this seafood place for it's safe food!

B DC Penn Quarter 801 Pennsylvania Ave NW, Washington, DC 20004 (202) 808-8720

Get great bourbon, beer and burgers with dedicated fryers and a dedicated gluten free kitchen space.

Chaia 3207 Grace St NW, Washington, DC 20007 (202) 333-5222

Gluten free beer and healthy food options in this Celiac-friendly place.

Wicked Waffle 1712 I St NW, Washington, DC 20006 (202) 944-2700

Dedicated kitchen space, waffle maker and amazing food!

Dedicated Gluten Free

Seoul Spice 145 N St NE #400, Washington, DC 20002 (202) 792-8879

Asian and dairy-free friendly, they serve my favorite bibimbap.

Il Canale 1065 31st St NW, Washington, DC 20007 (202) 337-4444

Gluten Free New York Pizza in DC.

Rise Bakery 2409 18th St NW, Washington, DC 20009 (202) 525-5204

Choose from a variety of delicious dedicated baked goods!

17
TRAVELING GLUTEN FREE IN NATIONAL PARKS

There really isn't a better way to learn about America's heritage than a National Park. National Park Week is held the last week of April every year. The National Park Service and the National Park Foundation have a big celebration for America's treasured places during National Park Week.

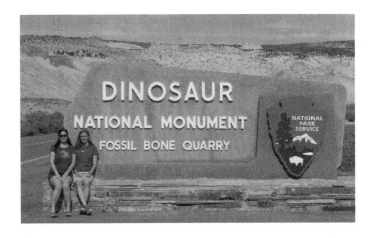

I moved to Utah to be close to five of the most amazing National Parks: Zion, Bryce, Capitol Reef, Canyonlands, and Arches. Every time I visit, no matter how many times I've been to each park, I'm in awe of the beauty of southern Utah's red rock country. The glow of the red rock is especially gorgeous against the vivid blue Utah sky. If you want to know more detail about the majestic parks Utah has to offer, check out my series of three podcasts on Utah National Parks Episodes #48, 49, and 51.

I always love visiting National Parks as there are so many activities to do, which is why they're one of my favorite places to travel. I've never gone to a National Park and have been disappointed. It doesn't matter if they're big or small, our National Parks are going to WOW you with each visit.

The most recent National Park I've been to is Devils Tower. Technically a National Monument, Devils Tower, is part of the National Park Service. Suppose you've ever seen the Stephen Spielberg flick Close Encounters of the Third Kind from the early 80s. In that case, you'll recognize this geologic feature as this is the place that aliens landed and communicated with humans in the movie.

Way before its recognition in pop culture, Devils Tower has been a sacred place to Native Americans living in the area for over a millennium. Today, you can see many colorful prayer flags that Native Americans leave at trees around the monument in traditional ceremonies. It's beautiful to see. I would highly recommend going to view the prayer ribbons and hike the two major trails around Devils Tower. It's a fantastic experience, and you'll have fond memories of your trip.

ANOTHER FAVORITE NATIONAL PARK area I visited with my friend and travel companion @SpanishNomad is in Virginia.

ELIKQITIE

We visited several Historical National Parks such as; Jamestown Settlement, and they were a blast. We learned so much information about American history, and we also learned about historical events that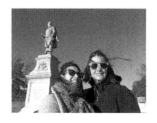
weren't taught correctly when we were in primary school. One event we learned new information about was the pilgrims at Plymouth Rock. In school, we were informed they were the first people to land in America. We learned from a Park Ranger that the settlers in Jamestown were actually the first people to settle in America from Europe.

NATIONAL PARK HISTORY

Today, we have over 1200 National Parks in our nation, but we started small. First, with Yellowstone, then adding more land and parks. When our country decided to put aside land for all to enjoy, we didn't even have park rangers or a park system!

To understand our National Park System, I'm also going to take you on a brief tour of the National Park Service website and the National Park Foundation.

To understand our National Park system's culture, you must go back in time and learn how the National Park system formed and the heritage of our National Parks. When first created, our National Parks weren't organized into an efficient system. Woodrow Wilson signed the first act on March 1st, 1872. Congress established Yellowstone National Park in the territories of Montana and Wyoming, "for the benefit and enjoyment of the people." With the founding of Yellowstone Park, our country started our National Park Movement.

Park management was delegated under the exclusive

control of the Secretary of the Interior. A new federal bureau in the Department of the Interior was responsible for protecting the 35 National parks and monuments that were to be established.

Before 1916, although our country had National Parks, they weren't part of a system, and they were left to be managed on an individual basis. Therefore, every park was managed entirely differently. Woodrow Wilson put them all in a system to be governed by the Federal Government. At this point, Park Rangers were hired to help protect our lands.

President Woodrow Wilson signed for the National Park Service so that the service established "should promote and regulate federal areas known as National Parks, Monuments and Reservations. And to conform to the fundamental purpose of the parks, which is to conserve the scenery and the natural, historic objects and the wildlife in the park and to provide for the enjoyment of people for generations."

In 1933, they transferred 56 National monuments and military sites from the Forest Service and the War Department to the National Park Service. This is the reason why our National Park Service isn't just parks! The NPS consists of National Monuments and National Historic Places as well.

WHY YOU MUST HAVE A NATIONAL PARK ANNUAL PASS

An annual park pass is $80, which covers everyone in your car for an entire year from the month your pass is bought. This is really a great deal because it usually costs between $15 and $25 for one carload of people to get into a park for one day. If you're going to a National Park for a few days and you want to see the entire park, get an Annual Park Pass because they're good all over the United States.

You can go to any National Park, historic monument, or a site in the United States with your Annual Park Pass. If you're a senior or in the military, you can get an Annual Park Pass for $55.

I purchase a new pass every year. However, make sure you keep your pass in a safe place because if you do lose it, they will not replace your pass. They don't have a computer system that keeps track of who owns a pass so you'll have to buy a new one. Even if you do have to buy a new pass, $160 for a whole family to go to multiple National Parks and participate in enjoyable outdoor activities is such a great deal. So, definitely get an annual pass, even if you go to four parks a year, it's totally worth it!

WHAT TO EXPECT WHEN YOU VISIT A NATIONAL PARK

When visiting a National Park, the entrance has a fun-sized cabin where National Park Rangers will greet you, take money for admission, and give you a map. They will also tell you of any significant closures before you go into the park. If you are using your Annual Pass, make sure to have your ID, as some rangers will ask you for identification.

Next, check out the Visitor Center, learn about the park, read the exhibits, see the movie, and look over the map to plan any hiking you want to do. Ask a ranger for assistance if you're not sure what hikes are suitable for your level and experience. Additionally, rangers will tell you if any of the trails are closed because of rockslides, nesting birds, or other activities going on in the park.

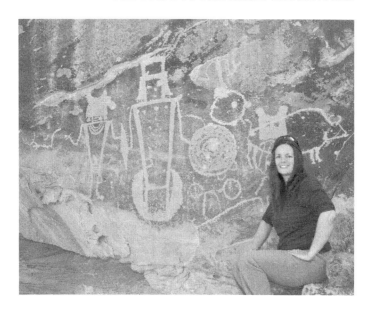

WHAT TO BRING AND HOW TO PACK FOR VISITING A NATIONAL PARK

Now, what do you want to pack when you go to a park? I can tell you from being Celiac, they're not going to have a lot of gluten-free choices if any. Definitely pack snacks and a lunch for whoever is gluten intolerant or has special dietary needs because they don't have a lot of safe food choices at parks. Many of the food vendors are also fast food, and they usually don't have staff that is trained for those of us with food allergies and dietary restrictions.

If you plan on going to a climate that is hot, like Utah in the summer, pack a water bladder and a backpack for each person. There are kid-sized water bladder and backpack combinations. I would recommend the Camelbak brand. I've had mine for 15 years and had only one small piece of plastic break off and replaced the bladder once. With a backpack and water bladder, you'll be hands-free to take pictures, and you don't have to worry about having enough water for each person. The guide for carrying water is to have 1.0 to 1.5 liters of water per adult and a half liter per child.

Also, you can refill your water bladder at the Visitor Center as many parks have a well pump located outside the main door. Usually, there aren't water fountains throughout the park, so make sure to have your water bladder filled before you go on your adventure! Always make sure to dump any leftover water from the day before to avoid germ buildup in your bladder. Additionally, when you are finished using your bladder, blow out the water in the straw, and let your bladder air out until it's completely dry. When your bladder is dry, crumple up paper towels and stuff your bladder so that any remaining water dries up and doesn't build mold or bacteria in your bladder.

Another benefit of having a backpack when you hike is that everybody has their own snacks, lunch, and jacket in their own bag. This process gives mom and dad from carrying kids' stuff. Water bladders with backpacks are a really convenient way to go when you're traveling, in a car, especially at National Parks. You can also put a small box or small cooler in the back of your vehicle with different flavored drinks such as Vitamin water, coconut water, and iced tea. Avoid drinks with dairy as they can spoil quickly in the heat.

Lastly, you can put your souvenirs, keys, and cell phone all in one place. Many bags have carabiner hooks so you can hook valuable items like your car keys so they won't get lost. I once lost my car keys in a pit toilet and had to fish them out! This is definitely an experience I will NEVER forget!

WEAR HIKING SHOES WHEN YOU'RE HIKING AT NATIONAL PARKS

I know you're probably wondering why I'm putting this information in my book. Here's the 411: I've seen people on trails in heels, flats, flip-flops, and other non-athletic type shoes. Yes, I seriously have seen this more times than I care to think about it! Make sure to wear sneakers, hiking shoes, or sandals that are made for hiking that are durable with a strap across your ankle.

In addition to good hiking shoes, make sure to avoid jeans, corduroy, and any clothing you don't want to get stained. Wear sweat-wicking material, as these are cooler and more comfortable than cotton. When hiking in Utah, dress in layers! The weather saying in Utah is: If you don't like the weather, wait 20 minutes! Also, as soon as the sun goes down, the temperature will drop 20 to 25 degrees in a matter of minutes. I realized this the first summer I lived in Utah. When the sun is out in Utah, it's sweltering. As soon as it sets, the heat index drops dramatically. You can feel the heat coming off of the rocks!

And if you're coming to Utah, it doesn't matter what season, always bring sunscreen! Many people make the mistake of not wearing sunscreen in the winter because it's cold. However, since Utah is at such a high elevation - many of the ski resorts between 7,000 and 9,000 feet at their peak - we are closer to the sun and receive more radiation and less atmospheric protection. In the wintertime, you get more than double the sun as you receive direct sunlight and also the sunlight bouncing off the sparkling white snow. You will burn much easier in Utah than in Florida!

I've seen skiers get a nasty sunburn on their face because they think, "Oh, it's cold, I won't get a sunburn." That is absolutely not true. Radiation does not care what the temperature is outside. Always bring and wear sunscreen, especially on your face, arms, and any part of your body that is exposed in Utah because you can quickly get sunburned.

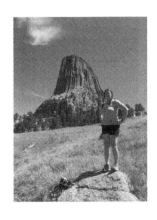

In addition to sunscreen, also bring sunglasses because the sun is really bright, especially at our high elevation. Many people wear sunglasses, even in the wintertime, as we have sunshine in Utah 300 days of the year!

ACTIVITIES TO DO IN A NATIONAL PARK

With so much to do at our National Parks, how can you decide what activities to schedule into your vacation? How should you navigate the park you choose to visit? What can you do in a National Park? What do you want to do? Find out about local geographic features? Maybe you want to learn about the history of our country's government or the history of the local area? You might be interested to learn about the ecosystem of the Everglades or finding out about the Native American cultures that first settled the region.

What you can do depends on the park you are going to visit. Many parks offer hiking, but some provide backcountry hiking, which usually requires a permit. If you're planning on going to a National Park, start at the National Park Service website at nps.gov. Once you get to the site, look at the tab on the left. This area will show you lodging options inside the park, activities, and if they have a Junior Ranger program for kids. These official park websites will also offer the latest updated information on what services and events are unavailable at the parks or activities that are closed due to COVID.

NAVIGATING THE NATIONAL PARK SERVICE WEBSITE

To find a park, land on the National Park Service page, and look for the little banner that says 'Find a park by the state". When I click on Utah, a map comes up informing me about the name and location of parks in Utah.

You can click on individual parks. Utah has 13 National Parks and almost 15 million visitors per year. This option shows the locations of parks on a map. Once you see all the parks and areas available, you can click on one specific park.

When I click on Arches, I have the option to sign-up for their newsletter. On the side, you can find the tab, "Plan your visit." From here, you can see opportunities for eating, lodging, hiking trails, things to do, and trip ideas. Also, find calendars, places to go, photos of the park, and park maps.

Download a pdf version of the map or look at the map online to see trail maps, view campsites, find the location of the Visitor's Center and activities throughout the park. In Arches, under the "Things to Do" tab, they have auto touring, backpacking, biking, canyoneering, commercial tours, hiking, Horseback riding, photography, ranger-led programs, rock climbing, and stargazing.

While many know about hiking in National Parks, there is so much more to do and see! Find an engaging activity, attend a ranger program or browse the gift shops.

JUNIOR RANGER PROGRAM

One of the best activities my kids loved to do at each of the National Parks is the Junior Ranger Program. Kids can get an activity guide from the Visitor's Center at no cost. When they complete the activities in the guide, bring their book back to the Visitor's Center, and your child will be "sworn in" as an Official Junior Ranger by a park ranger!

NATIONAL PARK PROGRAMS

Each park has different programs, depending on the location of the park and what the park has to offer. Park Rangers lead various programs such as stargazing, park history, geology, and nature programs. Programs are held at a different time each day and are usually posted outside the Visitor's Center. Some programs require you to sign-up, and others are more casual. Visit out the information desk to sign up for a program.

BACKCOUNTRY HIKING AND CAMPING

There are so many fantastic outdoor backcountry opportunities at National Parks; however, you may need a permit to access these adventures. Some areas have a limit on the number of days you can have a permit; others are only for day-use. Inquire about a backcountry permit as soon as you decide you would like a wilderness adventure as many of these permits are reserved months or weeks ahead of time. Few permits are given away the same morning you want to hike backcountry. Inquire from the information desk or on the National Park website ahead of time to find out details of the permit you would like to receive.

ASK A PARK RANGER

The Rangers are so knowledgeable, you can walk in up to the counter and tell them, "We have a family, we just want to experience easy hikes. What do you suggest?" Or "I love backcountry hikes, what do you suggest?" "What are some things I could get permits for?"

Park Rangers always have a suggestion, they're full of knowledge and know the ins and outs of the park. So, definitely ask a Ranger at the counter for tips on what you can do, they'll even circle or highlight information on your map, show you where to go and what to do. If you get to the park when the Visitor Center is open, definitely watch the movie before you venture off into the park because the video gives you the context of park culture.

SELF-GUIDED TOURS AT NATIONAL PARKS

Some parks have numbered spots where you can stop and do your own self-guided tour. So, if You can get out and view as many of them as you want, stay as long as you'd like or look for a couple minutes, get some pictures and hop back in the car.

Parks typically have one main loop around the main attractions and sites of the park. It's effortless to stop and see significant points of interest and scenery. You don't even have to hike when you visit a park. Simply stop at a pullout and take pictures. Warning: Utah parks during the summer are very crowded, and your chances of getting a spot at a pullout are rare if you are there during peak times. Go at 4pm or after to get a less crowded experience and good pictures at Utah's National parks.

Whatever you decide to do when you visit a National Park, please remember that our parks are here for our heritage! Make sure to recycle whenever possible and throw all trash in the proper containers. Also remember to take only photographs, not any of the geology of our parks so we can all enjoy the beauty of our parks for generations to come!

THE NATIONAL PARKS FOUNDATION

The National Park Foundation can be found at https://www.nationalparks.org and is a foundation that financially supports the National Parks. This foundation not only supports the National Parks, but they also have great information about special events happening at different parks around the country!

No matter what you love to do: explore the history, adventure in the outdoors, or find out about Native American culture, you will find something to love in our National Park System. Our system is unmatched across the world, which is why you'll hear so many different languages when you visit a park. We are incredibly fortunate to have this magnificent travel opportunity right in our own backyard!

18
TRAVEL ABROAD

When traveling outside the United States, you're adding more challenges to eating safely depending on where you have decided to vacation; however; you can overcome these issues and throw down the gluten-free gauntlet with the following overseas travel advice!

PASSPORTS AND PASSPORT ID

Just because you have a passport doesn't mean you can travel abroad! Did you know that some countries have a requirement that your passport needs to be valid at least 6 months after your date of travel? Also, some countries will accept your Passport ID as valid identification and others will need a regular passport. Check with the country you are traveling to, along with the expiration date of your passport to verify you can get into the country you are going to vacation. Also remember, that children's passports expire sooner than adult passports. Keep your passports updated and make sure that you have enough time on your passport so that it doesn't expire when you are traveling abroad.

PLACES TO VISIT ABROAD

With the entire world to visit, how does one decide where to go next? What should be on your bucket list? What country should you visit? Where should you go abroad for the first time? There are many questions you could be asking if you've never been outside the United States. The first time I traveled abroad was for my first honeymoon when my former husband and I went to Ixtapa, Mexico, for a week. Your first experience abroad will definitely be quite a culture shock if you visit another country that isn't a first-world country. Travel abroad gives you a sense of how small one person is on this vast big globe. When I visit another country, I also realize how humanity has the same basic wants in life - we are very different, yet, very similar in many ways to other people in different cultures.

WHAT COUNTRY SHOULD I VISIT FOR MY FIRST TRIP ABROAD?

When you're gluten-free, there are definitely experiences that will excite and inspire you. However, you may know from experience that finding food may not be so "inspirational," especially if you have more than one food you're trying to avoid.

In Episode #45, I interviewed Tarryn from My Celiac Life. We discussed traveling abroad gluten-free. Tarryn finds traveling abroad difficult. "I was always a big traveler before I was diagnosed, but still I'm quite a big traveler now, but it's something that you really have to look into, the language barrier, different options, bringing food everywhere you go, especially on trips. Plus, you have to be more open to those kinds of things just because we'll never know how long it will take to find something that you can eat, or you know, to feel comfortable in general."

"Then it's the idea of do they know the severity of Celiac, or do they think, this is something I'm choosing to do by choice. People don't always understand the severity. If I'm not sure if they understand properly, I'll either go with my gut or go home and make myself a sandwich." I'd say that's excellent advice because you can never be too safe when Celiac is eating at an unfamiliar restaurant speaking a foreign language.

Traveling abroad can bring many challenges, including, but not limited to, what to pack for your flight or cruise abroad, watching your liquid sizes, the types of foods you have access to that are safe at the location you are traveling to, and, the biggest challenge, the language barrier!

For your first overseas experience, I would definitely recommend trying out a country where many locals speak English, so you have less chance of being glutened. I'd also recommend flying to the country you want to visit and traveling via cruise, which lowers your chances of getting sick even more. You can easily skip eating lunch during the day when you are out galivanting around because of the sheer amount of food you will eat at other times during your cruise. Two of my favorites I would definitely recommend: London and Iceland.

ALWAYS CARRY FOOD WITH YOU IN YOUR BACKPACK

Even the most gluten-free savvy traveler can get stuck without safe food to eat - you miss your plane, or it's delayed, and now you're sitting in an airport overnight without food. When you wake up in the morning, you don't have many food choices. A myriad of craziness can always happen during your adventure that has nothing to do with being gluten-free and yet, affects us anyway! I'll give you advice on traveling overseas, along with information from gluten-free influencers from my podcast.

BETTER QUALITY FOOD IN LONDON AND EUROPE

Except for the plane ride, I'm always excited about traveling to and in Europe, especially when I think about the fantastic food I'm going to eat. The quality of food is much better, as many foods are locally sourced and fresh. Europe does not use GMO, and modified foods on the scale as we do in the US and factory farming isn't their mainstay for raising food. Because of these factors, Europe's food tastes better and has less of the chemicals and hormones we have in our diet.

I've heard from other Celiac that they can eat the dairy in Europe, but not the US. I have experienced the same. While I can eat imported dairy without issue, American dairy poses many digestive issues for my system.

MOST BEAUTIFUL PLACES IN THE WORLD TO VISIT

Out of the 12 countries I've visited, I'd say the most beautiful place to visit in Iceland. The second most beautiful place in the world, in my opinion, is Southern Utah. Both are similar; however, if you have been to Utah, Iceland is geologically similar to Utah. You would then need to add three-feet thick layers of moss, hot springs in every town, ponies, waterfalls and magical rainbows to the geology of Southern Utah to qualify as Iceland. It's insanely amazingly beautiful, and I've never heard anyone say a word different about this country.

UNIQUE COUNTRIES TO VISIT

Yes, Iceland is also on this list! I'd also add Austria to my "Unique Countries to Visit" list. I love the mix of city and rural areas, both of which are gorgeous. Vienna has a fantastic vibe, and the countryside is absolutely stunning. There's also the town of Innsbruck, steeped in over a millennium of history and culture. Additionally, there are many fun modern things to do in Innsbruck and an incredible train system to take you anywhere you want to go.

TOP TRAVEL DESTINATIONS IN THE WORLD

Fiji, Antarctica, and Iceland would be my top three destinations. Only as recently as 2019, visitors could forgo the transit across the bottom of South America by sea and fly directly from South America to Antarctica, which is a much better choice if you suffer from motion sickness. Additionally, you spend less time commuting to your destination and enjoying your trip if you fly.

Fiji looks like paradise and, although I haven't been to Fiji yet, this country has been on my bucket list for years. Flights to Fiji are the most significant cost factor to visit this beautiful country. Save up your money and place a picture of a hut on the ocean upon your vision board. Everyone I know that has gone to Fiji had only positive experiences in this small country.

If you take one trip out of the country your entire life, go to Iceland. Read more about Iceland on my Iceland page below and check out my fellow podcaster Danielle Desir's Nature, Nurture, and Adventure to plan your Iceland trip! Listen in to Episode #60, where Danielle talks about her Iceland experience, right before I left to go vacation in this beautiful country.

TOOLS YOU CAN USE WHEN DINING ABROAD

Even if the country you are visiting does not speak English, you can effectively navigate an international menu with the following tools. Having the right gluten-free tools is essential when eating during your travels. Three necessary tools, listed below, are critical to the success of your overseas trip. Remember, communication is vital and be proactive, ask questions, and do your best to make sure the wait staff understands your needs as a Celiac.

Gluten Free Dining Cards

Dining Cards are statements that you bring with you on 4 x 6 paper pieces that tell your server in their language that you're gluten-free. I'd be glad to send you a set of dining cards when you contact me through my website www.travelglutenfreepodcast.com

I've brought my own dining cards to different countries and have had decent success except France. For some reason, many restaurants in France don't understand why in the world anyone wouldn't want to eat gluten! I remember once handing my card to a maitre'D outside a restaurant, asking if he could accommodate me. His response? A resounding and loud, "No! We can't serve you any safe food here; you must go somewhere else to eat!" Of course, I didn't eat there, and this is a perfect example of why Paris and France in general, have a reputation for being rude to tourists.

Now, that being said, there are dedicated gluten-free bakeries and restaurants in Paris that you can feel safe eating at while in the "City of Romance." You'll want to visit Helmut Nutcake, the most amazing, dedicated gluten-free bakery in France when in France. I came home with a massive bag of gluten-free goodies!

THE GUIDE TO TRAVELING GLUTEN FREE

. . .

Contact Your Hotel, Resort or Airbnb Ahead of Your Trip

I'm a big plan-ahead person, and I always contact the resort or hotel I'm staying at ahead of time to find out what accommodations they have for gluten-free dining. Contact the resort or hotel you are visiting and let them know you have Celiac disease. Provide dining cards to both the wait staff and the individuals who are cooking the meals.

When looking for an Air, I'll always pay a bit more for a room with a fridge. This is hugely accommodating when you get dinner out and have leftovers, or you have that exotic chocolate you purchased that ended up a bit melty, and you need to chill it back to shape. Additionally, if you stay there for three days or more, you can stop by the grocery store and pick up a few necessities, such as non-dairy milk, to have chilled for a quick and easy protein drink in the morning.

Use the European Allergen Codex

European Allergen Codex is a system in which you can easily see what allergens are in restaurants' different foods. When you use this system, remember that they list the opposite of the US - where we show what foods you CAN eat, the European Allergen Codex shows which allergens are in the food. For example, if you see the letter "G" next to a food, it contains gluten and is NOT gluten-free.

They are created by the Labelling Directive from The European Food Safety Authority (EFSA). This authority decided on a commission, The Codex Alimentarius Commission, which agreed on foods to be included in The European Food Allergen Codex. This Codex is the allergen regulation standard used across Europe. While the Codex list contains the major allergens worldwide, the foods, which are common causes of allergic reactions, differ between geographical areas. As a result of dietary preferences. Depending on what foods are used by ethnicity, some countries have chosen to include new foods on their national list of possible allergens. The EU has decided to add celery, mustard, sesame seeds, lupin, and mollusks and products created from these foods as allergens.

The European Commission has recently published draft legislation that includes food safety culture. A recent revision for food hygiene also covers allergen management and redistribution of food. The Codex Alimentarius Commission is expected to adopt a revision of its standard on General Principles of Food Hygiene by the end of 2020. This update introduces the food safety culture to increase awareness and improve employee performance in eating establishments.

The update to the current CODEX introduces requirements on good hygiene practices to prevent and limit foods causing allergies or intolerances in equipment, processing, and storage in containers used for harvesting, transport, and storing food at the end destination.

This Codex is the same system across Europe's countries, which I have traveled, which is nice to worry about one less thing when you are eating while traveling. If the restaurant doesn't have the Codex Allergen list on their menu, as the Maitre'd, if they have an allergen menu, they may have a few copies of special menu allergens. Many restaurants I ate at in Europe were very accommodating and went out of their way to serve safe food.

BEST PLACES TO VISIT WHEN YOU ARE GLUTEN FREE

My top countries for gluten-free travel are England, Italy, Canada, and Iceland. I have specific reasons why I love each

THE GUIDE TO TRAVELING GLUTEN FREE

of these countries, and it's not only because of the fantastic food they have to offer.

Besides having fantastic gluten-free food in each of these places, there are many cultural, historic, and outdoor recreational pastimes these places have to offer. If the words ancient, historical, and city all describe a destination - I'm there. Also, I love thrill-seeking in the mountains, especially red rock and unusual geologic formations.

The following countries are listed in alphabetical order and contain highlights of each country. Although these are not an entire list of all countries I've visited, I wanted to include countries with the best foodie experiences for my gluten-free people! Who wants to go on vacation to a country that doesn't appreciate Celiac disease?

Australia

Many of us with Celiac disease and gluten intolerance RAVE about eating in Australia. Many restaurants are familiar with and accommodate gluten-free dishes. The Land Down Under is a great place to travel if you're gluten-free for several different reasons.

First, many places speak Aussie English, so you don't have to worry about the language barrier. That's a big hurdle out of the way when trying to eat safely. Secondly, grocery stores and other markets usually carry a selection of gluten-free foods to quickly stop and grab a safe bite to eat at a market if you can't find a restaurant.

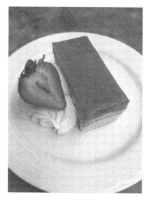

You will be able to find a variety of dedicated gluten-free

restaurants and many other places that are knowledgeable about food allergies. Use the methods listed in this book, do your research in advance, and have fun exploring Australia's city life.

CANADA

Home of Katz donuts, you can travel to almost any city in Canada and acquire amazing experiences plus phenomenal food. Canada is the only country I've been to with more dedicated fryers than London! Although many cities in Canada are gluten-free friendly, I'd recommend Victoria. Ellen Baynes of The Celiac Scene started the gluten-free movement in Victoria. Find out more details on Episode #21 of my podcast.

THE CANADIAN CELIAC ASSOCIATION

The Canadian Celiac Association does a great job of monitoring products that are safe for Celiac. The Canadian Celiac Association in Canada monitors a lot of different restaurants, and Canadians take their gluten-free seriously. This is easy to see in the amount and quality of restaurants you'll safely eat.

ENGLAND

The city of London has many gluten-free fryers and the quaintest family-owned markets with many organic and gluten-free food choices on every corner. Tons of museums, shopping, and take a big bus tour to see the different neighborhoods. I'll go into more detail on my London page and in The Guide to Traveling Gluten Free. Essentially, you can't go wrong with a trip to London.

THE GUIDE TO TRAVELING GLUTEN FREE

If you're interested in fun gluten-free food, London, England is the place you want to visit! You're bound to find gluten-free in many food ethnicities when perusing London restaurants. Like fried food? No worries! London is teeming with food establishments that have dedicated fryers. I've eaten more than my fair share of fried food while in London, and I believe you will too!

Want to eat a delicious gluten-free dessert from a dedicated gluten-free bakery? You'll find many dedicated bakeries, so eat pastries, doughnuts, and croissants to your heart's content - and remember to leave space in your luggage to bring home goodies you've acquired from your amazing London trip!

Jenny Finke and I talk about the fun we had in London and a few of the places we both loved to eat in Episode #72. Check out that episode for our fun chat on her stay and my visit to London.

Vegetarian and Vegan Options in London

My daughter Aliyah is Celiac and vegetarian, which offers yet another level or two of complexity when we eat out. In London, however, there are quite a few options for those who are both gluten-free and vegetarian or vegan. I've even come across vegetarian restaurants who offer many gluten-free options on their menu! There are many vegetarian and vegan options in general in London. Additionally, many restaurants also offer dairy-free!

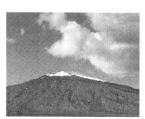

Iceland

Iceland is on the top of my list for geological formations. My first and only trip I visited Iceland on a cruise from London - a double bonus! I would definitely recommend this trip as I ate insane amounts of gluten-free bread and saw the most amazing sites. The next time I go to Iceland, I'm renting a van and hitting the Ring of Fire highway and taking a 360 around Iceland's edge.

You'll find lots of fish and meat; Iceland isn't very vegetarian friendly. The food is high-quality and delicious no matter where you go in Iceland. Iceland is one of the countries I can eat the dairy and actually drank a pint of chocolate milk in one sitting without feeling ill!

Italy

Italy sounds like the weirdest place to eat well because of all the pasta and bread. However, Italy has the highest per capita of Celiac cases in the world, which is why many places are Celiac-friendly. In a country where almost half of the population is Celiac, you'll need to offer safe food to stay in business! You'll be able to find amazing pastries, pizzas and pastas that are safe and gluten-free when traveling around Italy.

Norway

Visit the Bergen Fish Market for aisles upon aisles of fresh seafood caught on the shores of Norway! Get a reindeer or moose burger and choose from your choice of animal jerky including elk, reindeer and beef. There isn't a lack of fresh meat and fish in this northern country

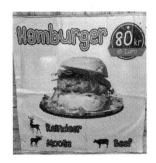

and their food is very fresh! Fair warning: the food is quite expensive so remember to budget accordingly.

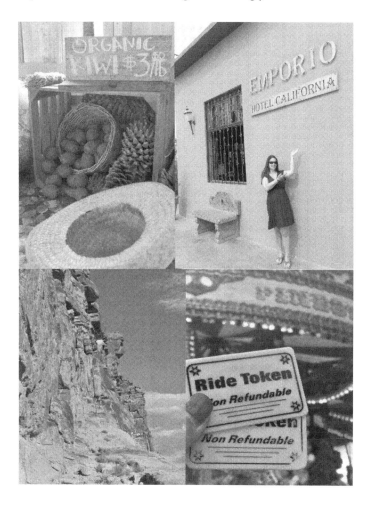

Chapter 01 | What is Gluten?
"What Is Gluten?" Celiac Disease Foundation. N.p., n.d. Web. https://celiac.org/gluten-free-living/what-is-gluten/

"Natures Legacy." Nature's Legacy. N.p., n.d. Web. 14 Aug. 2020. https://natureslegacyforlife.com/about/what-is-spelt

"Sources of Gluten." Celiac Disease Foundation. N.p., n.d. Web. 14 Aug. 2020. https://celiac.org/gluten-free-living/what-is-gluten/sources-of-gluten/

Chapter 02 | Certified Gluten Free and Gluten Free Foods
"Gluten Intolerance Group of North America." Gluten Intolerance Group of North America - Donations. N.p., 09 July 2020. Web. 14 Aug. 2020. Gluten-Free Certification Organization (GFCO)

Chapter 03 | The Challenge to Eating Out Gluten Free
"OpenTable." OpenTable. N.p., n.d. Web. 14 Aug. 2020. OpenTable

Find Me Gluten Free App. "Find Me Gluten Free App - Available for IOS and Android." Find Me Gluten Free App - Available for IOS and Android. N.p., n.d. Web. 15 Aug. 2020.

100% Gluten-Free App. "Dedicated Gluten Free Around the World App." For Gluten Sake. N.p., 02 Aug. 2019. Web. 15 Aug. 2020.

Tripadvisor. "Read Reviews, Compare Prices & Book." Tripadvisor. N.p., n.d. Web. 15 Aug. 2020.

Chapter 04 | How to Plan Ahead for Gluten Free Travel
TSA. "Travel Checklist." Travel Checklist | Transportation Security Administration. N.p., n.d. Web. 14 Aug. 2020. https://www.tsa.gov/travel/travel-tips/travel-checklist

Chapter 05 | Using Gluten Free Apps to Shop for Safe Food
"Celiac Disease Foundation." Celiac Disease Foundation. N.p., n.d. Web. 14 Aug. 2020. www.Celiac.org.

Makeena App. "Makeena: Healthy Savings - Apps on Google Play." Google. Google, n.d. Web. 15 Aug. 2020.

Schar gluten free app. "Schär Gluten Free - Apps on Google Play." Google. Google, n.d. Web. 15 Aug. 2020.

"Gluten Free Foods : Target." Bitly. N.p., n.d. Web. 14 Aug. 2020. https://bit.ly/39vNKR2

www.facebook.com/fearlessdining. "Ultimate Gluten Free Costco Shopping Guide: Printable Shopping List." Fearless Dining. N.p., 28 Dec. 2019. Web. 14 Aug. 2020. https://bit.ly/2CQZpyb

"Gluten Free Bakery - Bread, Donuts and Cookies." Safeway. N.p., n.d. Web. 14 Aug. 2020. https://bit.ly/32TKFJn

Heather, and Kayla. "Shopping at Kroger Gluten Free and Dairy Free." Gluten Free, the Bible, and Me. N.p., 24 Apr. 2019. Web. 14 Aug. 2020. https://bit.ly/2D4VaPd

"Gluten-Free Diet." Whole Foods Market. N.p., n.d. Web. 15 Aug. 2020. https://bit.ly/2EcGaiK

Chapter 08 | Supplements You Can Travel With When You're Gluten Free

"C. Difficile Infection." Mayo Clinic. Mayo Foundation for Medical Education and Research, 04 Jan. 2020. Web. 15 Aug. 2020. https://www.mayoclinic.org/diseases-conditions/c-difficile/symptoms-causes/syc-20351691

Parry, Wynne. "What's in Your Gut? 3 Bacterial Profiles Defined." LiveScience. Purch, 20 Apr. 2011. Web. 15 Aug. 2020. https://www.livescience.com/13810-gut-bacteria-metagenomics-digestive-symbionts.html

Chapter 12 | Travel By Air

"Travel Tips: 3-1-1 Liquids Rule: Transportation Security Administration." Travel Tips: 3-1-1 Liquids Rule | Transportation Security Administration. N.p., n.d. Web. 15 Aug. 2020. https://bit.ly/3g36bzf

"Top Rated Allergy-Friendly Airlines." SPOKIN. N.p., n.d. Web. 15 Aug. 2020. https://www.spokin.com/top-rated-airlines-peanut-free?_branch_match_id=692854221431188880

Delta Airlines Dietary offerings. (n.d.). Retrieved May 01, 2020, from https://www.delta.com/content/www/en_US/traveling-with-us/onboard-services/special-meals.html

Alaska Airlines. "Main Cabin Food and Drinks." *Alaska Airlines*, www.alaskaair.com/content/travel-info/flight-experience/main-cabin/airbus-food-and-drink.

Virgin Atlantic Specialised Meals | Dietary Requirements ... flywith.virginatlantic.com/gb/en/prepare-to-fly/dietary-requirements.html.

"Order a Meal for Specific Dietary Requirements." *Virgin Atlantic Specialised Meals | Dietary Requirements | Virgin Atlantic*, flywith.virginatlantic.com/gb/en/prepare-to-fly/dietary-requirements.html

JetBlue. N.p., n.d. Web. 15 Aug. 2020.

"In the Air." In the Air. N.p., n.d. Web. 15 Aug. 2020.

https://www.southwest.com/html/customer-service/inflight-experience/index.html

"Special Meals and Nut Allergies." - Travel Information - American Airlines. N.p., n.d. Web. 15 Aug. 2020. https://www.aa.com/i18n/travel-info/experience/dining/special-meals-and-nut-allergies.jsp

Lufthansa.com. N.p., n.d. Web. 15 Aug. 2020. https://www.lufthansa.com/us/en/Special-meals

"What Food and Drinks Does Spirit Offer on the Plane?" What Food and Drinks Does Spirit Offer on the Plane? · Spirit Airlines Support. N.p., n.d. Web. 15 Aug. 2020. https://customersupport.spirit.com/hc/en-us/articles/202097886-What-food-and-drinks-does-Spirit-offer-on-the-plane-

"Special Meals: Qatar Airways." Qatarairways.com. N.p., n.d. Web. 15 Aug. 2020. https://www.qatarairways.com/en/services-special/special-meals.html

7, Aug, Jun 5, and Feb 6. WOW Air. N.p., n.d. Web. 15 Aug. 2020. https://wowair.us/travel-info/service-board/meals-on-board/

"Dietary Requirements: Travel Information: Before You Fly: Emirates United

States." United States. N.p., n.d. Web. 15 Aug. 2020. https://www.emirates.com/us/english/before-you-fly/travel/dietary-requirements.aspx

Chapter 14 Camping
"Freeze Dried & Dehydrated Backpacking Food." Backpacker's Pantry. N.p., n.d. Web. 15 Aug. 2020.

"Dehydrated Camping Meals & Backpacking Food: Good To-Go®." Go. N.p., n.d. Web. 15 Aug. 2020.

"Freeze Dried Food." Mountain House. N.p., n.d. Web. 15 Aug. 2020.

"YETI Drinkware, Hard Coolers, Soft Coolers, Bags And More." YETI Drinkware, Hard Coolers, Soft Coolers, Bags And More. N.p., n.d. Web. 15 Aug. 2020.

"Backpacking Food: Freeze Dried & Dehydrated Meals: REI Co-op." REI. N.p., n.d. Web. 15 Aug. 2020.

"Meal Planning for Backpacking." REI Co-op. N.p., n.d. Web. 15 Aug. 2020. https://www.rei.com/learn/expert-advice/planning-menu.html

Chapter 15 Cruising Gluten Free
American Cruise Lines "Frequently Asked Questions." FAQ's & Important Passenger Information | American Cruise Lines. N.p., n.d. Web. 15 Aug. 2020

Argyll Cruise (Scottish) "Cruise the Scottish Islands: Argyll Cruising - Example Menu." Argyll Cruising. N.p., 18 July 2020. Web. 15 Aug. 2020. https://www.argyllcruising.com/life-on-board/example-menu/

Carnival Carnival Cruise Line. "Guests With Disabilities." Carnival Cruise Line. N.p., n.d. Web. 15 Aug. 2020. https://www.carnival.com/about-carnival/special-needs/dietary-needs.aspx

"Welcome to Celebrity Cruises: Modern Luxury Lives Here." Celebrity Cruises | Luxury Cruises, Cruise Deals & Vacations. N.p., n.d. Web. 15 Aug. 2020.

Crystalcruises.com. N.p., n.d. Web. 15 Aug. 2020.

Disneycruise.disney.go.com. N.p., n.d. Web. 15 Aug. 2020.

"Special Dietary Needs? It's Easy to Cruise with Holland America Line." Holland America Blog. N.p., 24 Jan. 2018. Web. 15 Aug. 2020.

Norwegian Coastal Express "What about Special Dietary Needs?" Frequently Asked Questions. N.p., n.d. Web. 15 Aug. 2020. https://www.ncl.com/it/en/cruise-faq/dietary-needs

Oceania Cruises https://www.oceaniacruises.com/experience/dining/

Pearl Seas Cruises Frequently Asked Cruising Questions Answered by Pearl Seas Cruises. N.p., n.d. Web. 15 Aug. 2020. https://www.pearlseascruises.com/frequently-asked-questions

Cruises, Princess. "Princess Cruises: FAQ: Cruise Answer Place : Dining & Nightlife." Www.princess.com. N.p., 09 Jan. 2020. Web. 15 Aug. 2020. https://www.princess.com/learn/faq_answer/onboard/dining_nightlife.jsp

Royal Caribbean. "What Options Are Available for Dietary Restrictions?: Royal Caribbean Cruises." What Options Are Available for Dietary Restrictions?| Royal Caribbean Cruises. N.p., n.d. Web. 15 Aug. 2020. https://www.royalcaribbean.com/faq/questions/dining-dietary-restrictions-customer-care

Viking Cruises. "Frequently Asked Questions: Viking River Cruises." Viking Cruises. N.p., n.d. Web. 15 Aug. 2020.
https://www.vikingrivercruises.com/frequently-asked-questions.html

Chapter 17 | Traveling Gluten Free in National Parks

National Park Service "NPS.gov Homepage (U.S. National Park Service)." National Parks Service. U.S. Department of the Interior, n.d. Web. 15 Aug. 2020.

WORK WITH ME

Wouldn't You Love Your Own Personal Gluten Free Travel Planner?

Love *The Guide to Traveling Gluten Free*? Would you like me to walk with you step-by-step in planning your next vacation as your personal gluten-free travel planner?

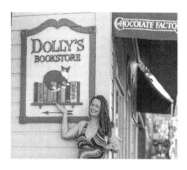

Contact me through my contact page on my website at http://www.travelglutenfreepodcast.com to inquire about Personal Travel Planning packages for your next trip!

SHARE THIS BOOK WITH THE WORLD!

I'd love to reach more of our gluten-free community and give them the freedom to travel safely!

By writing a recommendation for my book, The Guide to Traveling Gluten Free, you are giving other gluten-free friends who love to travel an opportunity to learn how they can be free of worry and food anxiety when planning their next vacation!

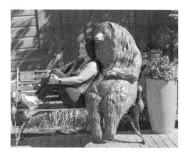

Share the love in *The Guide to Traveling Gluten Free* by leaving a book review!